REDEFINING MIDLIFE

The Modern Handbook for Embracing
Change & Empowering Your Life

By Matilda Anderson Ph.D

Copyright @ 2025 Matilda Anderson Ph.D

Disclaimer

This publication, *Redefining Midlife: The Modern Handbook for Embracing Change & Empowering Your Life*, is intended solely for educational and informational purposes. It is not a substitute for professional medical advice, diagnosis, or treatment. Before making any health-related decisions or changes to your healthcare plan, readers should consult qualified medical professionals.

While every effort has been made to ensure the accuracy and reliability of the information provided, the authors and publisher cannot guarantee its completeness or currency. Medical research is constantly evolving, and the content in this book may not reflect the most recent developments. The publisher and authors disclaim all liability for any errors, omissions, or outcomes that may result from the use of this information.

For specific health concerns or circumstances, readers are strongly encouraged to seek guidance from legal and medical professionals. By using *Redefining Midlife: The Modern Handbook for Embracing Change & Empowering Your Life*, you assume all risks associated with its content.

Legal Notice

All rights are reserved for *Redefining Midlife: The Modern Handbook for Embracing Change & Empowering Your Life*. The entire content is protected under copyright law. Except for brief quotations used for reviews or educational purposes, no part of this book may be reproduced, distributed, or transmitted in any form—whether by photocopy, recording, or other mechanical or electronic means—without the prior written consent of the publisher.

Any unauthorized reproduction or distribution of this work is strictly prohibited and may result in legal action. For inquiries or permission requests, please contact the publisher directly.

Table of Contents

Introduction 7
  Why This Book? 7
  How to Use This Guide 8

Chapter 1 12
Understanding the Journey 12
  Understanding Menopause and Perimenopause 12
    What is Perimenopause? 12
    What is Menopause? 13
    Why Do These Changes Happen? 14
  Why Do Perimenopause and Menopause Cause So Many Changes? 15

Chapter 2 22
Perimenopause – Early Signs and What to Expect 22
  What Is Perimenopause? 22
  Early Signs of Perimenopause 23
  Practical Tips for Managing Early Changes 25
  Embracing a New Chapter 27

Chapter 3 32
  Postmenopause – Living Well After the Change 32
  What Is Postmenopause? 32
  What Changes Might You Notice? 33
  Real-Life Inspiration: Carmen's Story 36
  Understanding Emotional Changes in Perimenopause and Menopause 37

    Bone Health and Physical Changes in Menopause 48

Chapter 4 51

    Nutrition and Exercise for Menopause Relief 51

    Herbal Remedies and Supplements—What You Need to Know 54

    The Role of Mind-Body Practices in Managing Menopausal Symptoms 57

Chapter 5 64

    Hormone Replacement Therapy (HRT) 64

        Alternative and Emerging Medical Treatments for Menopausal Symptoms 68

    Communicating Effectively with Healthcare Providers About Menopause 70

Chapter 6 77

    Real Stories, Real Strength – Navigating Perimenopause and Menopause 77

    Lessons Learned – Wisdom from Women Who've Been There 82

Chapter 7 89

    Building a Supportive Community During Menopause. 89

    How to Talk to Family and Friends About Menopause 97

Chapter 8 102

    Creating Your Personal Action Plan for Managing Menopause 102

    Monitoring the Effectiveness of Treatments and Lifestyle Changes 108

Chapter 9 115

Embracing the Changes of Menopause 115
    Understanding the Changes... 115
    Building a Support System 117
    Taking Action and Staying Positive 117
    Celebrating the Journey 118
Looking Forward: Embracing the Future with Optimism
.... 119

Introduction
Why This Book?

This book is essential because it offers a caring, all-in-one guide to understanding and managing the changes of perimenopause and menopause. It's written in clear, simple language so you don't need a medical background to understand it. Here's why it matters:

- **A Personal and Supportive Resource:**
  Menopause can feel overwhelming and isolating. This book provides personal stories and real-life experiences that show you're not alone. It offers encouragement and practical advice from women who have been through the same journey.

- **Educational and Easy to Understand:**
  Instead of using confusing medical jargon, the book explains what happens in your body in everyday language. It covers everything from the early signs of perimenopause to life after menopause, so you know what to expect and how to take care of yourself.

- **Practical Guidance for Everyday Life:**
  The purpose of the guide is to assist you in overcoming the difficulties caused by hormone flunctuation. It gives step-by-step advice on how to manage common symptoms like hot flashes, mood swings, and sleep issues. You'll find tips on nutrition, exercise, and self-care that you can easily incorporate into your daily routine.

- **Combining Natural Remedies and Medical Treatments:**
  Every woman's journey is unique. This book shows you how to blend natural remedies—like herbal supplements, yoga, and healthy eating—with medical treatments when needed. This balanced approach empowers you to choose what works best for your body and lifestyle.
- **Empowering and Reassuring:**
  The goal of the book is to turn a challenging time into an opportunity for growth and self-care. By understanding the changes in your body, you can embrace this new phase of life with confidence and a sense of control.

How to Use This Guide

In short, this book is your friendly, easy-to-follow companion on the journey through perimenopause and menopause. It offers clear explanations, practical tips, and heartfelt support to help you feel informed, empowered, and prepared for the changes ahead.

This guide is designed to be your easy-to-follow companion on your journey through perimenopause and menopause. Here's a simple, step-by-step explanation of how you can get the most out of it:

Start with the Introduction:
Begin by reading the introductory chapters. They explain why this book exists and how it can help you. These sections set the stage and let you know what to expect from the guide.

Understand the Journey:
The early chapters break down what perimenopause and menopause are, and explain the changes you might notice. This part uses everyday language, so you can easily understand the science behind the changes without feeling overwhelmed.

Explore the Stages:
The book is organized into sections for each stage—perimenopause, menopause, and postmenopause. Each section focuses on the specific challenges and changes of that phase. You can jump to the stage that matches your current experience, or read them in order to see the full picture.

Dive into Symptom Spotlights:
Specific symptoms like hot flashes, mood swings, sleep problems, and more are covered in their own chapters. Each section gives clear advice on both natural and medical options to help you manage these challenges. Use these chapters as a reference whenever you need focused guidance on a particular symptom.

Check Out Natural Remedies and Lifestyle Tips:
In the sections on nutrition, exercise, herbal remedies, and mind-body practices, you'll find practical tips that you can start using right away. These parts show you simple, everyday steps to help manage symptoms and boost your overall well-being.

Review Medical Treatments and Professional Guidance:
If you're considering treatments like Hormone Replacement Therapy or other medical options, these chapters offer balanced information. They also include tips on how to communicate with your healthcare provider, ensuring you feel confident discussing your needs.

Connect with Personal Stories:
Real-life experiences and inspirational journeys are shared throughout the book. These stories remind you that you are not alone and can offer practical lessons from others who have navigated this path.

Build Your Support Network:
Look for sections that focus on finding community and support from family and friends. These tips are designed to help you create a network that understands and supports your journey.

Create Your Personal Action Plan:
Use the guided steps provided to combine natural remedies with medical treatments in a way that suits your lifestyle. There are practical strategies for tracking your progress and adjusting your approach as needed.

Use the Resources Section:
At the end of the book, you'll find additional resources like recommended books, websites, and organizations. This section is a handy reference if you want to explore more detailed information or join supportive communities.

Tips for Navigating and Applying the Advice:

- **Read at Your Own Pace:**
  Don't feel pressured to read the book in one sitting. Take your time with each section and revisit parts as needed.
- **Take Notes:**
  Jot down tips or ideas that resonate with you. This can help you remember useful advice and apply it to your daily routine.
- **Apply One Change at a Time:**
  Try incorporating small adjustments based on the

advice, whether it's a new exercise, a dietary tip, or a relaxation technique. Gradually build your personal action plan.

- **Keep an Open Mind:**
Every woman's experience is unique. Use the suggestions as a starting point, and adapt them to what feels right for you.

By following these steps and tips, you'll be well-equipped to use this guide as a supportive, practical tool throughout your journey. Enjoy the process of learning and growing—this book is here to help you every step of the way.

Chapter 1

Understanding the Journey

Understanding Menopause and Perimenopause

Menopause is a natural stage in a woman's life when her periods stop for good. It usually happens between the ages of 45 and 55, but every woman is different. It's not a sudden event—it's a process that takes years, and it comes with changes in hormones that can cause different symptoms.

Before menopause, there is a stage called **perimenopause**. At this point, a woman's body begins to get ready for menopause. Some women barely notice it, while others experience noticeable symptoms.

Let's break down each stage so you can understand what's happening in your body.

What is Perimenopause?

Perimenopause means "around menopause." It can start as early as a woman's late 30s or early 40s. This stage can last anywhere from a few years to over a decade before menopause actually happens.

During perimenopause, your **hormone levels start to change**—especially **estrogen and progesterone**, the two main female hormones. Instead of staying steady, these hormones go up and down unpredictably. This can lead to symptoms such as:

- **Irregular periods** (shorter, longer, heavier, or lighter than usual)
- Night sweats and hot flashes, which are abrupt sensations of heat, perspiration, and flushing
  - Changes in mood, such as irritation, anxiety, or an unusually high level of emotion
  - Sleep issues, such as difficulty falling asleep or waking up in the middle of the night
- **Brain fog** (forgetfulness, trouble focusing, or feeling mentally "foggy")
- **Weight gain** (especially around the belly, even without big changes in diet or exercise)
- **Vaginal dryness** (which can cause discomfort during intimacy)
- **Lower sex drive** (feeling less interested in sex)

These symptoms can come and go, and their intensity varies for each woman. Some women barely notice them, while others find them challenging.

What is Menopause?

Menopause officially happens when **you have gone 12 full months without a period**. At this point, the ovaries stop releasing eggs, and estrogen levels drop significantly.

By the time you reach menopause, the symptoms from perimenopause may start to ease, but some may continue. You might still experience:

- Hot flashes and night sweats
- Vaginal dryness and discomfort
- Mood changes
- Difficulty sleeping
- Joint pain or stiffness
- Changes in skin and hair (dryness, thinning, or loss of elasticity)

Low estrogen levels following menopause can raise the risk of certain illnesses since estrogen has a preventive function in the body, including:

1. **Osteoporosis,** which makes bones weaker and more brittle.
2. **Heart disease** (estrogen helps protect the heart, so the risk increases after menopause)

This is why it's important to take care of your health by staying active, eating well, and considering treatment options if needed.

Why Do These Changes Happen?

The main reason for these changes is **hormones**—especially **estrogen and progesterone.** These hormones control your menstrual cycle and many other functions in your body, including mood, metabolism, and skin health.

- Unpredictable symptoms are caused by fluctuations in estrogen and progesterone levels during the perimenopause.

- **During menopause:** Estrogen levels **drop sharply**, which is why symptoms like hot flashes can be intense.
- **After menopause:** Hormone levels **remain low**, and the body adjusts to functioning without as much estrogen.

Menopause is not an illness—it's a natural transition. However, the symptoms can be frustrating or even overwhelming. The good news is that there are **many ways to manage** these changes, including lifestyle adjustments, natural remedies, and medical treatments.

This book will help you understand your body and give you the tools to handle menopause with confidence. You are not alone—millions of women go through this, and with the right information and support, you can feel your best at every stage.

Why Do Perimenopause and Menopause Cause So Many Changes?

Menopause is not just about periods stopping—it's about how **hormones** affect almost every part of the body. The physical and emotional changes during **perimenopause** and **menopause** happen because of shifts in hormone levels, especially **estrogen** and **progesterone**.

To understand this better, think of hormones as **messengers** in your body. They tell different organs what to do. During perimenopause and menopause, these messengers start acting unpredictably, leading to symptoms like hot flashes, mood swings, and sleep problems.

Let's break it down step by step.

1. The Role of Estrogen and Progesterone

The two most important female hormones are:

- **Estrogen:** This hormone helps control your menstrual cycle and affects your brain, heart, bones, skin, and more. It keeps your body balanced and functioning smoothly.
- **Progesterone:** This hormone works alongside estrogen to regulate your cycle and help with sleep and mood. It also helps prepare the body for pregnancy.

During perimenopause, these two hormones start to **fluctuate**—going up and down unpredictably—before they eventually **drop to very low levels** after menopause.

Think of it like a **rollercoaster:**

- In your younger years, hormone levels are like a smooth, steady road.
- During perimenopause, the rollercoaster starts—hormones rise and fall sharply, leading to unpredictable symptoms.
- After menopause, the rollercoaster slows down, and hormone levels settle at a much lower level.

2. Why Do These Changes Cause Symptoms?

Since hormones affect so many parts of the body, their ups and downs during perimenopause can create a wide range of symptoms. Here's how it works:

Hot Flashes and Night Sweats

- Estrogen helps regulate the **body's thermostat** in the brain. When estrogen levels drop suddenly, the brain can get confused and think you're overheating.
- As a result, it **triggers a hot flash**—your blood vessels widen, making you feel a sudden wave of heat.
- At night, this can cause **night sweats**, making it hard to sleep.

Analogy: Imagine your thermostat at home starts malfunctioning, randomly blasting heat even when it's not needed. That's what happens inside your body during hot flashes.

Mood Swings and Anxiety

- Estrogen influences brain chemicals like **serotonin** and **dopamine**, which help regulate mood.
- When estrogen levels swing up and down, so do these brain chemicals—leading to mood changes, irritability, or anxiety.
- Some women feel fine one moment and overwhelmed the next.

Analogy: It's like your brain's "happy hormones" are on a seesaw—sometimes up, sometimes down, making emotions feel unpredictable.

Sleep Problems

- Progesterone helps you fall asleep because it has a natural soothing effect.
- When progesterone levels drop, it can lead to **restless sleep, waking up at night, or difficulty falling asleep**.
- Hot flashes and night sweats can also wake you up multiple times, making sleep even worse.

Analogy: Imagine trying to sleep while someone keeps turning the lights on and off—that's what's happening inside your body with hormone changes.

Brain Fog and Forgetfulness

- Estrogen plays a role in **memory and focus**.
- When estrogen levels drop, some women experience **brain fog**, forgetfulness, or difficulty concentrating.

Analogy: It's like trying to use a computer with too many programs open at once—your brain feels slower and harder to navigate.

Weight Gain and Metabolism Changes

- Estrogen helps regulate how the body **stores fat** and burns energy.
- Lower estrogen levels can lead to **weight gain, especially around the belly**, even if you're eating and exercising the same way as before.

Analogy: Think of your metabolism as a fire that used to burn brightly. With lower estrogen, the fire burns more slowly, so you store more fuel (fat) instead of burning it off quickly.

Vaginal Dryness and Lower Libido

- Estrogen keeps the **vaginal tissue** healthy and lubricated. When estrogen drops, the tissue becomes **thinner, drier, and less elastic**, which can cause discomfort during intimacy.
- Lower estrogen can also reduce **blood flow to the area**, leading to decreased sensitivity and libido.

Analogy: It's like a rubber band that has dried out—it becomes less stretchy and more fragile.

Weaker Bones (Osteoporosis Risk)

- Estrogen helps keep bones **strong and dense**.
- When estrogen levels fall, bones **lose density faster**, increasing the risk of fractures and osteoporosis.

Analogy: Think of bones as a sturdy wooden bridge. Without regular maintenance (estrogen), the wood starts to weaken and break more easily.

Higher Risk of Heart Disease

- Estrogen helps **protect the heart** by keeping blood vessels flexible and maintaining healthy cholesterol levels.
- After menopause, the risk of **high blood pressure, high cholesterol, and heart disease** increases.

Analogy: It's like losing the protective coating on your car—over time, the parts wear out faster without that extra layer of protection.

3. What Happens After Menopause?

Once you reach menopause (12 months without a period), hormone levels stabilize at **a much lower level.** While certain symptoms—like hot flashes—may get better with time, others—like bone loss and heart health risks—need ongoing care.

The key to feeling your best is **learning how to manage these changes**—whether through lifestyle adjustments, natural remedies, or medical treatments.

*Menopause is a transition, not an ending. Your body is adjusting to a **new normal**, and while the changes can be challenging, they don't have to control your life.*

By understanding the science behind these shifts, you can:
Recognize why symptoms happen *(so they don't feel scary or confusing)*
Learn how to manage them *(through lifestyle, natural remedies, or medical treatments)*
Take control of your health *(so you feel confident and strong during this stage of life)*

You are not alone in this journey, and with the right knowledge, you can navigate menopause with **confidence, comfort, and control.**

Chapter 2

Perimenopause — Early Signs and What to Expect

Perimenopause is the **first phase** of the menopause journey. It's like the body slowly turning the dial down on your monthly cycle—not all at once, but in waves over time. Many women aren't even aware they've entered this stage. That's because the changes are **gradual**, and the signs can sometimes be mistaken for stress, aging, or even other health issues.

Let's walk through this stage together so you can recognize the signs, understand what's happening in your body, and start making changes that will support you during this transition.

What Is Perimenopause?

The word "peri" means **around** or **near**—so perimenopause means "around menopause." It's the **lead-up phase** before your periods stop completely.

Most women enter perimenopause sometime in their **40s**, but it can start as early as the **mid-30s**. This stage can last for **several years**—sometimes up to 10—before menopause officially begins (which is when you've gone **12 full months** without a period).

The two primary hormones that control your monthly cycle, estrogen and progesterone, start to be produced less often by your body during the perimenopause. These hormones don't decline in a straight line. Instead, they go up and down unpredictably, which is why you might feel fine one day and off-balance the next.

Early Signs of Perimenopause

Not every woman will experience all of these symptoms, and the intensity can vary from person to person. But here are **some of the most common early signs:**

1. Irregular Periods

- Periods may come earlier or later than usual.
- You might skip a month or two, then suddenly have a heavier period.
- Flow can become lighter or much heavier than before.

Think of it like your body losing its rhythm—your cycle becomes unpredictable.

2. Mood Swings and Irritability

- You may feel more emotional, short-tempered, or easily overwhelmed.
- Anxiety or sadness might show up, even if nothing specific is wrong.

Some women describe it as feeling like a teenager again— moody without knowing why.

3. Hot Flashes or Night Sweats

- A sudden wave of heat spreads through your body, especially your chest, neck, and face.
- During the night, you may wake up soaked in perspiration.
  Your internal thermostat seems to be malfunctioning.

4. Trouble Sleeping

- You might have a hard time falling asleep or wake up often during the night.
- Even when you sleep, you may not feel rested.

5. Fatigue

- You may feel low on energy, even after sleeping well.
- Everyday tasks might feel more tiring than before.

6. Brain Fog and Forgetfulness

- You may forget names or misplace things more often.
- Concentration and focus can become harder.

7. Changes in Sex Drive

- You might feel less interested in sex.
- Vaginal dryness or discomfort may make intimacy difficult or less enjoyable.

8. Weight Gain or Body Changes

- Many women notice weight gain, especially around the belly.
- Your body shape may shift, even if you haven't changed how you eat or move.

Practical Tips for Managing Early Changes

The good news is that there are **many ways to ease the discomforts** of perimenopause. Here are simple lifestyle tips you can try:

1. Track Your Symptoms

Use a journal or an app to track your cycle, mood, sleep, and symptoms. This helps you notice patterns and prepare for changes.

2. Support Your Sleep

- Stick to a calming bedtime routine.
- Avoid caffeine late in the day.
- Keep your bedroom cool and dark.

Tip: Try chamomile tea or a warm bath before bed.

3. Move Your Body Daily

Exercise helps balance mood, reduce hot flashes, and support sleep. Yoga, dancing, and walking all count, so you don't need a gym!

Even 20-30 minutes a day can make a big difference.

4. Eat Nourishing Foods
- Eat more entire foods, such as fruits, vegetables, lean meats, and healthy fats.
- Reduce sugar and processed foods—they can make symptoms worse.
- Drink plenty of water to stay hydrated.

Try adding more leafy greens and foods rich in calcium and magnesium.

5. Practice Stress Relief

Hormone changes can make you more sensitive to stress. Try calming activities like:

- Deep breathing
- Meditation
- Gentle stretching
- Journaling or creative hobbies

Even 10 minutes a day can help reset your nervous system.

6. Talk to Someone

You're not alone. Speak with a trusted friend, a support group, or a healthcare provider. There's strength in asking for help and sharing what you're going through.

Real-Life Example: Maria's Story
The 42-year-old Maria began experiencing irregular periods and became extremely irritable with her children and

workplace. She also saw that she was sweating when she woke up and that her sleep was less restful. She initially assumed it was simply work-related stress. After reading more about perimenopause, she began tracking her symptoms and made small changes—like taking evening walks, eating more vegetables, and using a fan by her bed. She also spoke to her doctor about her mood swings and was reassured that what she was feeling was common.

Now, she feels more in control and better prepared for what's ahead.

A Gentle Reminder

Perimenopause can feel confusing or frustrating, but remember: **this is a natural stage of life**, not a sign of something wrong with you. Your body is doing what it's meant to do. With the right tools and knowledge, you can move through this transition with grace and strength.

This chapter is just the beginning. The rest of this guide will walk you through everything from hormone changes to natural remedies and medical options. But for now, take a deep breath, be kind to yourself, and know that **you're not alone**.

Embracing a New Chapter

Menopause is a **natural life transition**, just like puberty, pregnancy, or aging. But unlike those other changes, menopause often doesn't come with much guidance or support. Many women feel surprised, confused, or even scared when they reach this stage—but it doesn't have to be that way.

In this chapter, we'll explain what menopause really is, the key changes that happen in your body and mind, and how to move through this phase with confidence and calm. You'll also hear from real women who have navigated menopause in their own way—and come out stronger.

♀ Embracing Menopause with Confidence

Yes, this stage can be challenging—but it's also an opportunity for **renewal**. With the right mindset, tools, and support, menopause can be a **powerful turning point** in your life.

Here are some ways to manage this phase and feel more like yourself again:

1. Educate Yourself

The more you understand what's happening, the less scary it feels. Learning about your body gives you power. This book is here to walk with you through that.

2. Prioritize Sleep and Rest

Your body is adjusting to big hormonal changes. Rest is essential.

- Try a calming bedtime routine.
- Keep your bedroom cool.
- Limit screen time before bed.
- Reduce caffeine and alcohol, especially in the evening.

---

3. Nourish Your Body

Food is fuel and medicine. Aim for:

- Fresh vegetables and fruits.
- Whole grains.
- Lean proteins (like fish, eggs, beans).
- Healthy fats (like olive oil, nuts, and avocado).
- Calcium-rich foods to protect bones.

Drink water throughout the day to stay hydrated.

---

4. Stay Active

Movement supports mood, sleep, weight, and bone strength.

- Walking, swimming, dancing, or yoga can all help.
- You don't need a gym. Just get your body moving daily.

Even 20 minutes makes a difference.

5. Protect Your Mental Health

- Talk to friends, a therapist, or a menopause support group.
- Journal your thoughts.
- Practice deep breathing or mindfulness.
- • Ask for help when you need it—this is not a sign of weakness.

---

6. Examine Medical and Natural Alternatives
Numerous medical and natural cures are included in this book. You'll discover how to make the best decision for you based on your particular needs, whether that means using herbal teas, supplements, hormone therapy, or lifestyle modifications.
Consult your physician before beginning any new treatment.

Real-Life Inspiration: Helen's Story

Helen, age 54, reached menopause at 51. At first, she struggled with sleep problems, night sweats, and mood swings. She felt out of control and didn't know where to turn.

After reading about menopause, Helen started walking every morning, cut back on sugar, and joined a local women's support group. Her doctor helped her explore treatment options, and she chose a combination of herbal supplements and low-dose hormone therapy.

Now, Helen says, "Menopause taught me to put myself first—for the first time in my life. I feel stronger and more peaceful than I ever expected."

Menopause is not an ending—it's a beginning. It's a time to pause, reflect, and reclaim your health, energy, and identity. Yes, it can be uncomfortable at times, but it's also a chance to listen to your body and give it the care it truly deserves.

You are not broken. You are becoming.

This chapter is part of your toolkit. In the rest of this guide, we'll explore treatments, nutrition, mindset shifts, and more, so you can design a life that feels vibrant and free—even during big changes.

You've got this. And we've got you.

Chapter 3
Postmenopause – Living Well After the Change

Many women think the journey ends after menopause—but that's not true. In fact, **postmenopause** is a whole new chapter, and with the right care, it can be a time of strength, freedom, and renewed energy.

In this chapter, we'll explore what postmenopause means, what changes to expect, how to care for your body and mind long-term, and how to keep thriving in this next phase of life.

What Is Postmenopause?

Postmenopause is the **time after menopause**—when you've gone a full year without a period, and your hormone levels have settled into their new pattern.

This stage **lasts for the rest of your life.** Your ovaries no longer release eggs, and estrogen and progesterone levels stay low. Some menopause symptoms may fade away, while others might continue.

The good news? Many women report feeling **more emotionally balanced, confident, and self-assured** in this stage than ever before.

What Changes Might You Notice?

Every woman is different, but here are some things you might experience after menopause:

Lingering Symptoms

- Some women still have **hot flashes or night sweats**, though they're usually less intense.
- **Vaginal dryness** may continue, due to low estrogen.
- **Sleep issues or mood swings** can persist, especially if untreated earlier.

Mental Clarity Returns

Many women say that after the fog of perimenopause and menopause lifts, they feel **mentally clearer** and more focused.

Weight and Metabolism

It might be easier to gain weight now, especially around the belly. Your metabolism naturally slows down. But with healthy habits, this can be managed.

Why Long-Term Health Matters

After menopause, your body needs some **extra care** to stay strong and healthy for the years ahead. Here's why:

1. Bone Health

Estrogen helps protect bones. Without it, **your bones can become thinner**, leading to a higher risk of osteoporosis.

What helps:

- Eat foods rich in **calcium and vitamin D** (like leafy greens, dairy, fish).
- **Weight-bearing exercises** like walking or light strength training.
- Bone checks as recommended by your doctor.

---

2. Heart Health

Estrogen also supports heart health. The risk of heart disease increases after menopause.

Some strategies to reduce this risk include:

• Eating heart-healthy foods (fruits, vegetables, and healthy fats);

• Staying active;

• Reducing alcohol and smoking; and

• Managing blood pressure and cholesterol with your doctor's assistance.

---

3. Brain Health

Memory and focus can be affected during menopause, but staying **mentally active** helps long-term.

What helps:

- Read, do puzzles, or learn something new.
- Stay socially connected.
- Get enough sleep and manage stress.

4. Maintaining a Healthy Weight

Hormones and aging can make it easier to gain weight—but losing it is still possible with small changes.

What helps:

- Eat smaller portions, more often.
- Choose real, whole foods over processed snacks.
- Get some exercise each day, even if it's just a quick stroll.

♀ Lifestyle Tips to Feel Your Best

Here are simple changes that can make a big difference:

✅ Keep a Routine

A regular sleep schedule, meals, and exercise routine help your body stay balanced.

Stay Open to Treatment

Some women benefit from **hormone therapy** or **natural supplements** to manage ongoing symptoms. Talk with a healthcare provider to find what's right for you.

Stay Connected

Talk with friends, join a women's circle, or share your story. You're not alone. Support from others helps you feel heard and understood.

Real-Life Inspiration: Carmen's Story

Carmen, 57, thought life after menopause would be boring. She had gained weight, felt sluggish, and wasn't sleeping well. But she decided to take small steps—walking in the mornings, swapping soda for water, and going to bed earlier.

She also began journaling and practicing deep breathing to manage stress. After a few months, she felt lighter—physically and emotionally. She declared, "I'm not trying to be who I was at thirty." "I'm attempting to be my best self right now."

Getting Along After Menopause

This is your opportunity to prioritize yourself. Many women take on goals they had previously put off, travel, change employment, or pick up new interests. Your time has come, and you have earned your wisdom.

Here's what thriving looks like in postmenopause:

- **Confidence in your body**—knowing what it needs.
- **Freedom from periods, birth control, and pregnancy worries.**

- **Clarity in your priorities**—choosing what matters most.
- **Power in your voice**—speaking up for your needs.

Postmenopause is not the end of your story—it's a **new beginning**. With a little care, curiosity, and courage, you can continue living a full, vibrant life.

Understanding Emotional Changes in Perimenopause and Menopause

During perimenopause and menopause, many women experience emotional ups and downs. These changes are real, valid, and completely normal. You're not imagining things—and you're not alone.

Why Emotions Change

Hormones like estrogen and progesterone don't just affect the body. They also impact how we feel. As these hormones rise and fall, they can influence brain chemicals like serotonin, which helps regulate mood.

This can lead to:

- Mood swings

- Irritability
- Anxiety
- Sadness or low mood
- Feeling overwhelmed or more sensitive than usual
- "I just don't feel like myself," several women say. That's alright, this phase is a significant change. But feeling better can be achieved in a variety of ways.

Coping Mechanisms That May Be Beneficial

1. Recognize Your Emotions

Permit yourself to experience your emotions. Just acknowledge your feelings without passing judgment. This relieves stress and enables you to treat yourself with kindness.

2. Practice Self-Care

- Take breaks when needed.
- Spend time in nature or in quiet spaces.
- Enjoy things that make you laugh or feel calm, like music or hobbies.

3. Talk It Out

Talk to a friend, partner, or support group. Sharing how you feel can lift a huge weight. You may find others are going through the same thing.

4. Move Your Body

Even light exercise like walking or gentle yoga helps release feel-good chemicals and reduce anxiety.

5. Seek Professional Support

If emotions feel too heavy to handle alone, therapy or counseling can offer guidance. You can also speak to your doctor about treatments for depression or anxiety if needed.

Final Words of Support

Emotional changes are part of the journey—but they don't have to take over your life. Be patient with yourself, show yourself compassion, and remember—you're going through something big, and you're doing your best.

Sleep Disturbances During Menopause

Sleep is essential for feeling good and staying healthy. But during menopause, getting good sleep can become more difficult.

Why Sleep Gets Disrupted

Several changes during perimenopause and menopause can affect sleep:

- **Hot flashes or night sweats** wake you up suddenly.
- **Hormone shifts** (like lower estrogen) can make it harder to fall or stay asleep.
- **Mood changes** like anxiety or sadness can keep your mind racing at night.
- **Bladder issues** may wake you to use the bathroom more often.

Natural Sleep Aids

Try these gentle, drug-free remedies:

- **Chamomile tea or valerian root** before bed
- **Magnesium supplements**, with a doctor's guidance
- **Lavender essential oil** (on your pillow or in a diffuser)
- **Deep breathing or meditation** to calm the mind

Medical Options

If natural approaches aren't enough, speak to your doctor about:

- **Hormone replacement therapy (HRT)** for hot flashes and insomnia
- **Sleep aids** (short-term use only)
- **Melatonin supplements** to support natural sleep rhythms

Tips for Better Sleep

- Stick to a **regular bedtime and wake time**, even on weekends.
- Avoid screens (phones, TV) at least **30 minutes before bed.**
- Keep the room **cool and dark.**
- Limit **caffeine** and heavy meals in the evening.
- If you wake in the night, try **reading or listening to soothing music** instead of scrolling your phone.

Encouragement

You're not "bad at sleeping." Your body is changing, and it may take time to adjust. Be kind to yourself and know that better sleep is possible with the right tools and support.

Weight, Metabolism, and Menopause

Many women notice their body changing during menopause—especially around the belly. You may gain weight even if your eating habits haven't changed. It's frustrating, but it's not your fault.

Why Does This Happen?

- **Hormonal shifts**—Lower estrogen can lead to more belly fat and muscle loss.
- **Slower metabolism**—The body burns calories more slowly.
- **Less movement or sleep**—Fatigue and sleep problems can reduce activity and affect hunger hormones.

Nutrition Tips That Work

You don't need a strict diet—just smart choices:

Eat More:

- **Whole grains** (like brown rice, oats)

- **Vegetables and fruits**
- **Healthy fats** (like olive oil, avocado)
- **Lean protein** (chicken, beans, tofu)

Eat Less:

- Processed snacks
- Sugary drinks
- Fried or greasy foods

Drink plenty of **water**, and try not to skip meals—this helps with cravings and energy.

Exercise That Supports Hormone Health

You don't need to do intense workouts. Start small and stay consistent:

- **Brisk walking** (20-30 minutes a day)
- **Strength training** (2-3 times a week to keep muscles strong)
- **Stretching or yoga** for flexibility and calm

Even dancing in the kitchen counts—movement matters.

Lifestyle Shifts That Help

• Get enough sleep, as it aids in mood and hunger regulation.

• Control stress: a high level of tension makes it more difficult to control weight.

• Gently monitor your progress—not just on the scale, but also on how you feel.

Example: Lisa's Simple Routine

Lisa, 52, started walking her dog every morning and switched her sugary cereal for oatmeal with fruit. She also joined a fun dance class once a week. Over three months, she had more energy, slept better, and felt stronger—even though her weight barely changed.

"It wasn't just about the number," she said. "I just feel more like me again."

Vaginal and Sexual Health During Menopause

As women move through menopause, many experience changes in vaginal and sexual health. These changes are normal and nothing to be ashamed of—but they can be frustrating or confusing. The good news is, there are many ways to stay comfortable and feel confident again.

What Happens and Why?

As estrogen levels drop during menopause, the tissues in the vagina become:

- **Thinner**
- **Drier**
- **Less stretchy**

This can cause:

- Vaginal dryness
- Itching or burning
- Pain or discomfort during sex
- Less natural lubrication
- Changes in desire or arousal

These symptoms may affect how you feel about intimacy, your body, or your relationshp—but you are not alone, and you deserve to feel good in your body.

Medical Treatments That Can Help

1. **Vaginal Estrogen**
    - Comes as a cream, tablet, or ring
    - Helps restore moisture and thickness to vaginal tissues
    - Acts locally (stays in the vagina), with minimal hormone absorption
2. **Hormone Therapy (HRT)**
    - Systemic (whole-body) treatment for those with multiple menopause symptoms
    - Helps with vaginal changes and other issues like hot flashes
3. **Prescription Moisturizers or Lubricants**
    - Longer-lasting than regular lubricants
    - Use regularly to prevent dryness

Natural Remedies and Supportive Tips

- **Use Water-Based Lubricants:** Apply before and during sex to reduce discomfort.

- **Regular Sexual Activity or Vaginal Stimulation:** Helps keep blood flowing to the area and keeps tissues healthy.
- **Stay Hydrated and Eat Healthy Fats:** Drink water and eat foods like avocados, olive oil, and nuts to support tissue health.
- **Try Coconut Oil or Aloe Vera Gel:** Natural options some women use for light relief (always patch-test and consult a doctor first).

Emotional and Relationship Considerations

Changes in intimacy can be hard to talk about—but they're worth discussing. A loving partner will want to understand what you're going through. Open, honest conversations can deepen connection.

And if you're feeling unsure or anxious about these changes, consider speaking with a menopause-informed therapist or counselor.

You deserve to feel comfortable and confident in your body, no matter your age. These changes are natural—and with the right support and care, you can feel empowered and fulfilled in your sexual and personal well-being.

Brain Fog and Focus—Cognitive Changes in Menopause

Have you ever entered a room and forgotten your purpose? Or lose your train of thought mid-sentence? You're not alone—many women going through menopause experience what's often called "brain fog."

What's Going On?

Estrogen helps support brain function. When levels drop during perimenopause and menopause, it can affect how clearly you think or how well you remember things. This can cause:

- Forgetfulness
- Trouble focusing
- Feeling mentally "foggy" or scattered
- Slower thinking

These changes are usually temporary—but they can still be frustrating.

Tips to Boost Brain Health and Focus
1. Write It Down

Use notes, lists, or phone reminders. Keeping thoughts organized helps free up your mental space.

2. Get Moving

Exercise increases blood flow to the brain. A brisk 20-minute walk can sharpen thinking and lift your mood.

3. Stay Social

Talking with others helps keep the brain active and supports emotional health.

4. Prioritize Sleep

Sleep is when your brain resets and repairs. Aim for a consistent sleep schedule.

5. Eat Brain-Friendly Foods

- Berries
- Leafy greens
- Fatty fish (like salmon)
- Nuts and seeds
- Whole grains

These support memory and overall brain function.

Medical and Natural Options

- **Hormone Replacement Therapy (HRT)** may improve memory and focus in some women, especially during early menopause.
- **Supplements** like omega-3s, magnesium, or B vitamins might help, but talk to your doctor first.

- **Mindfulness or Meditation:** Even 5-10 minutes a day can improve focus and reduce stress.

⚡ Final Words

You're adapting to a significant change in your life, not going crazy. These brain changes are common and manageable. With small steps, you can feel clearer, more focused, and back in control.

Bone Health and Physical Changes in Menopause

Menopause doesn't just change how you feel—it can also affect your body's strength and structure. One important concern? Your bones.

Why Bone Health Matters

Estrogen helps keep bones strong. When it decreases, bones may become thinner or weaker, leading to a higher risk of osteoporosis (a condition that causes bones to break more easily).

Signs and Risks

Most women don't notice weak bones until they break one. That's why prevention is key. Risk factors include:

- Family history of osteoporosis
- Low calcium or vitamin D
- Not enough weight-bearing exercise

- Smoking or heavy alcohol use

How to Protect Your Bones
1. Exercise Regularly

- **Weight-bearing activities** like walking, dancing, or hiking keep bones strong.
- **Strength training** builds muscle and supports bones (e.g., lifting light weights or using resistance bands).
- **Balance exercises** like yoga reduce your risk of falls.

2. Eat Bone-Friendly Foods

Include:

- **Calcium-rich foods** like dairy, leafy greens, tofu, and fortified plant milks
- **Vitamin D** from sunlight, fatty fish, or supplements (helps the body absorb calcium)
- **Protein** to build and repair tissues

3. Get Regular Checkups

Ask your doctor about bone density tests (especially after age 50) to track your bone health.

Medical Support

- **Calcium and Vitamin D Supplements** if your diet doesn't provide enough
- **Prescription medications** (like bisphosphonates) to slow bone loss

- **Hormone Therapy (HRT)** may help protect bones during early menopause

Managing Other Physical Changes

You might also notice:

- Less muscle tone
- Changes in posture
- Joint aches or stiffness

These are common but manageable. Stay active, stretch daily, and get enough rest. Use hot packs or gentle movement to ease sore joints.

Your body is strong—and with a little care, it can stay that way. You don't need to do everything perfectly. Just take steady steps to move, nourish, and protect your body. You've come this far, and you're still growing stronger.

Chapter 4
Nutrition and Exercise for Menopause Relief

One of the best ways to feel better during menopause is by eating well and staying active. Food and movement can ease many symptoms like hot flashes, weight gain, mood swings, and sleep problems. This chapter will show you how to use nutrition and exercise to support your body through this transition.

Why Nutrition Matters

As estrogen levels drop, your body changes. You might:

- Gain weight more easily
- Lose muscle
- Feel more tired
- Crave unhealthy foods

But with the right meals, you can feel stronger, more energized, and more balanced.

Foods That Help

1. Calcium-Rich Foods For strong bones:

- Low-fat milk or yogurt
- Cheese
- Leafy greens (like spinach and kale)

- Fortified plant milks (soy, almond, oat)

2. Vitamin D Helps your body use calcium:

- Fatty fish (like salmon or sardines)
- Eggs
- Mushrooms
- A little sunlight on your skin each day

3. Protein To keep your muscles and energy strong:

- Chicken, turkey, fish
- Beans and lentils
- Tofu or tempeh
- Eggs and Greek yogurt

4. Whole Grains and Fiber Helps with digestion and keeps you full:

- Brown rice, oats, whole wheat bread
- Fruits like apples, berries, and pears
- Vegetables like carrots, broccoli, and sweet potatoes

5. Healthy Fats Good for your heart and hormones:

- Avocados
- Olive oil
- Nuts and seeds (especially flaxseeds and chia)

Foods to Cut Back On

- **Sugar:** Can make hot flashes worse and cause energy crashes.

- **Caffeine and spicy foods:** Might trigger hot flashes or night sweats.
- **Alcohol:** Can affect your sleep and mood.

Sample Daily Meal Ideas

Breakfast consists of oatmeal, fruit, and flaxseeds.
Lunch consists of quinoa, grilled salmon, and steamed spinach.
Snack: A handful of almonds and an apple
Dinner: Stir-fried tofu with vegetables and brown rice
Dessert: A small square of dark chocolate and herbal tea

Exercise: Move to Feel Better

Exercise helps with:

- Weight control
- Bone strength
- Better mood
- Sleep improvement
- Fewer hot flashes

Start where you are; a gym is not necessary.

Simple Weekly Exercise Plan

Day	Activity
Monday	30-minute brisk walk
Tuesday	Light strength training (resistance bands or water bottles)

Day	Activity
Wednesday	Stretching or gentle yoga
Thursday	Walk or dance at home
Friday	Strength training again
Saturday	Bike ride or swim (optional)
Sunday	Rest or light walk

Start small—just 10 minutes a day can make a difference. Find what you enjoy, and build up slowly.

Final Word

Your body is changing, but it's not giving up on you. With healthy food and regular movement, you can feel more in control, stronger, and even more confident than before. Small changes really do add up.

Herbal Remedies and Supplements— What You Need to Know

Many women are curious about natural remedies for menopause symptoms. Herbs and supplements can sometimes help—but they aren't always the right choice for everyone. This chapter will help you understand what works, what to be careful about, and when to talk to your doctor.

What Are Herbal Remedies?

Herbal remedies come from plants and have been used for centuries. They can be found in teas, capsules, tablets, or extracts.

Common Herbal Remedies and How They May Help

1. Black Cohosh
Often used for hot flashes and mood swings. Some women find relief, but others don't feel much difference.

2. Red Clover
May help with mild hot flashes. It contains plant estrogens (called phytoestrogens), which act like a weaker form of natural estrogen.

3. Dong Quai (Chinese Angelica)
Used in traditional Chinese medicine for hormone balance. Be cautious—may interact with medications or increase bleeding.

4. Evening Primrose Oil
Some use it for breast tenderness or mood swings. Research is mixed.

5. Maca Root
May help boost energy and mood. Found in powder or capsule form.

6. Flaxseed
Rich in omega-3s and plant estrogens. May help with mild hot flashes and supports heart and hormone health.

Supplements for Menopause Support

1. Vitamin D and Calcium
Essential for bone health after estrogen drops.

2. Magnesium
Can help with sleep, anxiety, and muscle cramps.

3. B Vitamins
Support energy and mood—especially B6 and B12.

4. Omega-3 Fatty Acids
Good for your heart, brain, and mood.

Important Warnings
Natural doesn't always mean safe. Certain plants may have adverse effects or interact with medications.
Read labels at all times. Make use of reputable products with quality assurance.
- Before beginning any supplement regimen, see your physician or pharmacist, particularly if you are on medication or have a medical condition.

When to Use Medical Advice Instead
- If your symptoms are severe or interfere with your day-to-day activities
- If, after a few months, natural therapies don't work; • If you feel worse or have strange adverse effects

- If you're unsure whether a product is safe

Sometimes, medical treatments like hormone therapy or antidepressants may be more effective—or safer for your situation. It's okay to combine natural remedies with medical care under your doctor's guidance.

Herbs and supplements can be helpful tools—but they're not magic cures. What works for one woman may not work for another. Be kind to yourself, stay informed, and remember: the goal is to feel better and thrive—your way.

The Role of Mind-Body Practices in Managing Menopausal Symptoms

Menopause brings many physical changes, but it also affects your emotions, stress levels, and mental well-being. One powerful way to manage these changes is through mind-body practices like yoga, meditation, and relaxation techniques. These practices help you stay calm, reduce stress, and support your physical health. In this chapter, we'll explore how these practices can help you feel better and how you can start using them in your daily life.

Why Mind-Body Practices Matter During Menopause

During menopause, your body is going through hormonal changes that can cause hot flashes, sleep problems, and mood swings. These changes can also bring stress, anxiety, and even feelings of sadness or overwhelm. This is where mind-body practices come in—they are gentle, natural ways to support your body and mind through this time.

Mind-body practices help in several ways:

- **Reduce stress and anxiety:** They encourage relaxation, which helps reduce stress hormones in the body.
- **Improve sleep:** Relaxation techniques can help calm your mind and body, making it easier to fall asleep.
- **Ease physical symptoms:** Practices like yoga and deep breathing can help relieve hot flashes, joint pain, and muscle tension.
- **Boost mood:** Mind-body practices can improve your mood and give you a sense of control during a time when you may feel like things are out of balance.

Yoga: Movement for Mind and Body

Yoga is a fantastic mind-body practice that combines gentle movement, breathing exercises, and relaxation techniques. It can be especially helpful during menopause because it helps manage stress, improves flexibility, and supports hormonal balance.

Benefits of Yoga for Menopause:

- **Reduces Hot Flashes**: Some studies show that regular yoga can reduce the frequency and severity of hot flashes.
- **Improves Sleep**: Yoga relaxes the nervous system, which can help with insomnia.
- **Relieves Joint Pain**: Many women experience joint pain or stiffness during menopause. Yoga stretches can help keep the body flexible and reduce discomfort.
- **Boosts Mood**: Yoga helps release endorphins (the "feel-good" hormones), which can improve mood and reduce anxiety.

Simple Yoga Poses to Try:

- **Cat-Cow Pose (Marjaryasana-Bitilasana)**: A gentle flow between two positions that stretches the spine and helps release tension in the back and neck.
- **Child's Pose (Balasana)**: A resting pose that calms the mind, reduces stress, and stretches the lower back.
- **Tree Pose (Vrksasana)**: A balancing pose that helps improve focus and calm the nervous system.
- **Downward-Facing Dog (Adho Mukha Svanasana)**: A full-body stretch that helps relieve tension in the body and boost circulation.

Meditation: Calm Your Mind

Meditation is the practice of sitting quietly and focusing your mind. It can help reduce the stress and anxiety that often come with menopause. Even just a few minutes of meditation each day can make a big difference in how you feel.

Benefits of Meditation for Menopause:

- **Reduces Stress**: Meditation helps you relax, which lowers the levels of stress hormones in your body.
- **Improves Focus**: It trains your mind to focus, which can help with memory and concentration.
- **Enhances Sleep**: Meditation helps calm the nervous system, making it easier to fall asleep and stay asleep.
- **Lifts Mood**: Regular meditation can improve your overall sense of well-being, reduce feelings of anxiety, and help you manage emotions.

Simple Meditation Techniques:

- **Mindfulness Meditation:** Sit quietly and focus on your breath. Pay attention to the sensation of the air moving in and out of your body. When your mind starts to wander, gently bring your focus back to your breath.
- **Guided Meditation:** Use a recorded meditation that leads you through a visualization, relaxing your body and mind step by step. There are many apps and websites offering guided meditations specifically for stress and menopause.
- **Body Scan Meditation:** Close your eyes and focus on each part of your body, starting from your toes and moving up to your head. Notice any tension and breathe into that area to release it.

Breathing Techniques: Relax and Refresh

Deep breathing exercises can help calm your mind and relieve stress. When you focus on your breath, it signals to your body that it's time to relax.

Benefits of Breathing Techniques:

- **Reduces Anxiety**: Deep breathing helps slow down your heart rate and reduces anxiety.
- **Eases Hot Flashes**: Slow, deep breaths can help reduce the intensity of hot flashes and provide relief.
- **Improves Focus**: Breathing exercises increase oxygen flow to the brain, which can improve concentration.
- **Calms the Nervous System**: Deep breathing helps activate your body's relaxation response, reducing stress and tension.

Simple Breathing Techniques to Try:

- **4-7-8 Breathing**: Inhale for 4 seconds, hold your breath for 7 seconds, and exhale for 8 seconds. Repeat several times.
- **Abdominal Breathing**: Place one hand on your chest and one on your stomach. Breathe deeply, allowing your belly to rise as you inhale and fall as you exhale. This helps slow your heart rate and calm your mind.
- **Alternate Nostril Breathing**: Close one nostril with your finger and inhale deeply through the other nostril. Switch and exhale through the opposite nostril. This technique helps balance the body and reduce stress.

Progressive Muscle Relaxation (PMR): Release Tension

Progressive muscle relaxation is a technique where you tense and then release each muscle group in your body. It's a great way to unwind and release any physical tension.

Benefits of PMR:

- **Reduces Muscle Tension:** Helps release the tightness that can come with stress or hot flashes.
- **Improves Sleep:** Relaxing the body before bed can make it easier to fall asleep.
- **Reduces Anxiety:** The physical relaxation helps calm your mind and reduce feelings of nervousness or restlessness.

How to Do PMR:

1. Find a quiet place to sit or lie down.
2. Start with your feet—tighten the muscles for 5 seconds, then relax them for 10 seconds.
3. Move up your body—legs, abdomen, chest, arms, neck, and face—repeating the same process.
4. Focus on how the muscles feel when relaxed.

Incorporating Mind-Body Practices into Your Life

The key to benefiting from mind-body practices is consistency. Start by choosing one or two practices and try to do them every day.

Practical Tips for Daily Practice

- **Start Small:** Begin with just 5 minutes of yoga, meditation, or breathing exercises. Gradually increase the time as it feels comfortable.
- **Make It Part of Your Routine:** Try to do your practice at the same time every day—whether it's in the morning to start your day or at night to relax before bed.
- **Find Support:** Join a yoga class or meditation group (in person or online) to stay motivated and connect with others who are going through similar experiences.
- **Be Patient with Yourself:** It can take time to feel the full benefits of these practices. Be kind to yourself and celebrate the small wins.

Mind-body practices can be a powerful tool to help you navigate menopause with more ease and balance. Whether you're looking for relief from hot flashes, better sleep, or improved mood, yoga, meditation, and relaxation techniques can help. Start small, stay consistent, and remember: you're in control of how you feel, and these practices are here to support you.

Chapter 5
Hormone Replacement Therapy (HRT)

Hormone Replacement Therapy (HRT) is a medical treatment used to help manage the symptoms of menopause. As the name suggests, HRT replaces hormones that your body no longer produces in sufficient amounts after menopause, specifically estrogen and progesterone. This can help reduce symptoms like hot flashes, night sweats, mood changes, and vaginal dryness. In this chapter, we'll look at what HRT is, its benefits and risks, and who might consider using it.

What is Hormone Replacement Therapy (HRT)?

As women enter menopause, their bodies naturally produce less estrogen and progesterone, which can cause a variety of symptoms. HRT works by replacing these hormones to restore balance, helping to ease symptoms.

There are two main types of HRT:

- **Estrogen-only HRT:** This is typically used for women who have had a hysterectomy (removal of the uterus).
- **Combined HRT (Estrogen and Progesterone):** This is used for women who still have their uterus. The combination of estrogen and progesterone helps

prevent the risk of uterine cancer, which can be a concern if estrogen is taken alone.

HRT can come in several forms, including:

- **Pills:** Taken daily, they are the most common form of HRT.
- **Patches:** These are applied to the skin and release hormones over time.
- **Gels and creams:** Applied to the skin.
- **Injections:** Less common, but still an option for some women.

Benefits of Hormone Replacement Therapy (HRT)

HRT can offer significant relief from menopausal symptoms. Some of the key benefits include:

- **Relieves Hot Flashes:** Hot flashes, one of the most common symptoms of menopause, can be greatly reduced with HRT. Estrogen helps regulate body temperature, reducing the intensity and frequency of these sudden heat surges.
- **Improves Sleep:** Many women experience sleep disturbances during menopause, especially due to hot flashes or night sweats. HRT can help alleviate these issues, leading to better, more restful sleep.
- **Reduces Vaginal Dryness:** Low estrogen levels can cause vaginal dryness, leading to discomfort during sex. HRT helps restore moisture, improving sexual health and comfort.
- **Prevents Bone Loss:** Estrogen plays a key role in bone health. Taking HRT can help prevent bone

thinning (osteoporosis), reducing the risk of fractures.
- **Improves Mood:** Some women experience mood swings, irritability, or even depression during menopause. HRT can help stabilize mood by balancing hormone levels.
- **Supports Heart Health:** Estrogen has a protective effect on the heart. For some women, HRT may help reduce the risk of heart disease after menopause.

Risks of Hormone Replacement Therapy (HRT)

While HRT has many benefits, it's important to be aware of potential risks. These risks vary depending on the type of HRT, the duration of use, and individual health factors.

- **Breast Cancer:** For women using combined HRT (estrogen and progesterone), studies have shown a slight increase in the risk of breast cancer with long-term use.
- **Blood Clots:** HRT, especially in pill form, may increase the risk of blood clots. Women who smoke, are overweight, or have a history of blood clots may be at higher risk.
- **Stroke:** Some studies suggest that long-term use of HRT may increase the risk of stroke, particularly in women who start HRT later in life.
- **Uterine Cancer:** For women who still have their uterus, taking estrogen alone can increase the risk of uterine cancer. This is why combined HRT is typically recommended.
- **Gallbladder Disease:** Some studies suggest that HRT may increase the risk of gallstones or other gallbladder problems.

Who Might Consider HRT?

HRT is not right for everyone, but it can be an excellent choice for women who:

- Have moderate to severe menopausal symptoms (like hot flashes, night sweats, or vaginal dryness).
- Are under 60 or within 10 years of menopause, as studies show that starting HRT early may have the most benefits.
- Have a family history of osteoporosis or other conditions that can benefit from HRT, such as heart disease or bone loss.
- Want a more effective option than lifestyle changes or other treatments for managing their symptoms.

However, HRT may not be suitable for women who:

- Have a history of breast cancer or certain types of hormone-sensitive cancers.
- Have a history of blood clots, stroke, or heart disease.
- Are at a higher risk for certain conditions due to factors like smoking, being overweight, or being over 60.

It's essential to have a discussion with your doctor to weigh the benefits and risks of HRT based on your personal health history and preferences.

Alternative and Emerging Medical Treatments for Menopausal Symptoms

In addition to HRT, there are other medical treatments that can help manage menopausal symptoms. Some of these treatments are more recent or are options for women who cannot take HRT. Let's take a look at some of the most common alternatives.

1. Non-Hormonal Medications

These medications do not replace hormones, but they can help manage some symptoms of menopause.

- **Antidepressants (SSRIs and SNRIs):** These medications can help alleviate mood swings, anxiety, and depression. Some have also been shown to reduce hot flashes.
- **Gabapentin:** Originally used to treat seizures, gabapentin has been found to reduce the frequency and severity of hot flashes, especially at night.
- **Clonidine:** Typically used for high blood pressure, clonidine can help reduce hot flashes in some women.
- **Vaginal Moisturizers and Lubricants:** For vaginal dryness, non-hormonal moisturizers and lubricants can provide relief during sex and help maintain vaginal health.

2. Selective Estrogen Receptor Modulators (SERMs)

SERMs are a type of medication that can mimic estrogen in some parts of the body while blocking it in others. They are sometimes used to help protect bone health, particularly for women who can't take traditional HRT.

3. Bioidentical Hormones

Bioidentical hormones are compounds that are chemically identical to the hormones your body produces. These hormones can be prescribed to address menopause symptoms and are available in various forms, including creams, patches, and pills. Some women prefer bioidentical hormones because they are marketed as being more natural, though they are not necessarily safer than traditional HRT. It's important to work with a doctor to ensure they are used safely.

4. Alternative Therapies

While not as well-studied as medical treatments, some women find relief from menopausal symptoms through alternative therapies. These might include:

- **Acupuncture:** Used to help manage hot flashes, stress, and sleep problems.
- **Herbal Remedies:** Some herbs, like black cohosh or evening primrose oil, are believed to reduce symptoms. However, their effectiveness and safety

are still under research, and they should be used with caution.

HRT is a highly effective option for many women experiencing menopause symptoms. It offers relief from common symptoms like hot flashes, night sweats, and vaginal dryness, while also providing long-term benefits for bone health and heart health. However, it's not without risks, and it's important to consider these when making your decision. For those who may not be candidates for HRT, other treatments like antidepressants, gabapentin, or alternative therapies may be helpful. Always talk to your doctor to discuss the best approach for your health and symptoms.

Communicating Effectively with Healthcare Providers About Menopause

Navigating menopause can feel overwhelming, and one of the most important steps in feeling empowered during this transition is to communicate clearly and effectively with your healthcare provider. Whether you're dealing with hot flashes, mood swings, or other menopausal symptoms, it's essential to have open, honest conversations with your doctor to ensure you get the care and support you need.

In this chapter, we will guide you through how to prepare for appointments, ask the right questions, and discuss both natural and medical treatment options, so you can feel confident in your healthcare decisions.

1. Preparing for Your Appointment

The first step in having an effective conversation with your healthcare provider is preparation. You don't have to walk into the office unprepared; taking some time beforehand can make a huge difference.

Keep a Symptom Journal

Track your symptoms before your appointment. This helps you remember what you've been experiencing, how often the symptoms occur, and how they affect your daily life. You can jot down things like:

- **Hot flashes**: How often they happen, how severe they are, and if they interfere with your daily activities.
- **Sleep problems**: Are you waking up frequently? Do you feel rested?
- **Mood changes**: Are you feeling more anxious, sad, or irritable than usual?
- **Other symptoms**: Any vaginal dryness, weight changes, or memory concerns.

Having this journal will give your healthcare provider a clearer picture of what you're experiencing, and help them make more informed recommendations.

Make a List of Your Medications

Include any over-the-counter supplements, vitamins, and herbs you are taking in addition to prescribed medications. Some natural remedies may interact with medical treatments, so it's important for your healthcare provider to know everything you are using.

Know Your Health History

Prepare to discuss any personal or family medical history that could impact your menopause care. For example, if you have a history of breast cancer, blood clots, or osteoporosis in your family, this could influence what treatment options are best for you.

2. Asking the Right Questions

It's easy to leave an appointment feeling unsure about what was discussed. To make the most of your time with your healthcare provider, ask specific, clear questions. Here are some examples of helpful questions to ask during your visit:

Questions About Symptoms:

- "Can you explain what's happening with my hormones and why I'm experiencing these symptoms?"
- "Are these symptoms normal, or should I be concerned about something else?"
- "What lifestyle changes can I make to help manage my symptoms?"

Questions About Treatment Options:

- "What are my treatment options for managing hot flashes, night sweats, or mood changes?"
- "Can you explain the benefits and risks of Hormone Replacement Therapy (HRT)?"
- "What are the alternatives to HRT, and how effective are they?"
- "What about natural remedies like herbs or supplements—are they safe to try, and do they actually work?"

Questions About Long-Term Health:

- "How can I protect my bone health during menopause?"
- "Should I be concerned about heart disease or other long-term health risks?"
- "How can I ensure I'm getting the nutrients I need as my metabolism changes?"

Questions About Side Effects and Risks:

- "What are the potential side effects of the treatment options you're recommending?"
- "How will I know if the treatment is working for me?"
- "How long will I need to be on medication, and when can I expect my symptoms to improve?"

3. Discussing Natural and Medical Treatment Options

It's common to be curious about both natural and medical treatments, especially when it comes to managing menopause.

Many women want to try natural remedies like herbs or lifestyle changes before turning to prescription medications. Here's how to approach these discussions with your healthcare provider.

Natural Treatment Options

Natural remedies can offer relief for some menopausal symptoms, but it's important to discuss them with your doctor before starting anything. Some common options include:

- **Herbs:** Black cohosh, red clover, and evening primrose oil are some herbs commonly used for managing hot flashes and mood swings.
- **Supplements:** Vitamins such as vitamin E, magnesium, and omega-3 fatty acids are sometimes used to help manage symptoms like mood changes and sleep disturbances.
- **Dietary Changes:** Eating a balanced diet rich in whole foods, fruits, vegetables, and healthy fats can support hormone balance and improve overall health.
- **Exercise:** Regular physical activity like walking, yoga, or swimming can help improve mood, maintain a healthy weight, and reduce hot flashes.

Medical Treatment Options

While many women prefer natural treatments, sometimes symptoms are severe enough that medical treatment is necessary. Some common medical treatments include:

- **Hormone Replacement Therapy (HRT):** This is often the most effective option for alleviating symptoms like hot flashes, night sweats, and vaginal

dryness. Your healthcare provider can help determine if HRT is right for you and explain the different types.
- **Non-Hormonal Medications:** If HRT isn't right for you, medications like antidepressants, gabapentin, or clonidine can help manage hot flashes and mood changes.
- **Vaginal Estrogen:** For women experiencing vaginal dryness, vaginal estrogen creams or suppositories can offer relief.

Don't hesitate to ask about both natural and medical options, and how they can work together. For example, your healthcare provider might suggest a combination of HRT and certain lifestyle changes to improve your overall well-being.

4. Being Honest and Open

It's essential to be open and honest with your healthcare provider about what you're experiencing, how you feel, and what you're hoping to achieve. This will help them create a treatment plan that suits your needs and preferences. If you're feeling unsure about a treatment option, express your concerns. It's okay to ask for more information or to seek a second opinion.

If you're considering alternative treatments, such as herbal supplements, let your doctor know. Some herbs or supplements can interact with medications, so it's important to be transparent. Your healthcare provider can help you navigate these options safely.

5. Follow-Up Appointments

Managing menopause often requires ongoing adjustments. If your initial treatment plan isn't working or if new symptoms develop, make sure to schedule follow-up appointments. Your healthcare provider can help adjust your plan as needed, and they can offer new treatments or suggestions as your body changes.

---

6. Trusting Yourself

Finally, trust your instincts. You know your body better than anyone else. If something doesn't feel right, whether it's a treatment or a recommendation, don't be afraid to speak up. You deserve to feel heard and supported throughout this journey.

Effective communication with your healthcare provider is key to managing menopause. By preparing ahead of time, asking the right questions, and discussing both natural and medical treatment options, you can feel confident in your healthcare decisions. Remember, you don't have to go through this transition alone. Your doctor is there to guide you, but you are the expert on your own body. Together, you can create a plan that helps you navigate menopause with ease and confidence.

Chapter 6
Real Stories, Real Strength - Navigating Perimenopause and Menopause

Menopause is a shared experience for all women, but no two journeys are the same. Every woman's path through perimenopause, menopause, and beyond comes with its own unique challenges and triumphs. The good news is that these challenges can be met with strength, resilience, and a great deal of support from others who have walked this path before. In this chapter, we will share stories of women who have faced their menopause transitions with courage and creativity. Their experiences can serve as inspiration and a reminder that you're not alone in this journey.

These are real stories from women who have navigated menopause successfully—each with their own set of struggles and victories. We hope these stories help you feel supported, empowered, and motivated to take control of your own experience.

1. Sarah's Story: Embracing Change with Confidence

Sarah, 52, had always been healthy and active, so when her periods became irregular and she started experiencing hot flashes, she was surprised. But what caught her off guard the most was how emotionally intense things became.

"I felt like I was losing control of my emotions," Sarah says. "One minute, I'd be fine, and the next, I'd burst into tears or get angry over the smallest things. It was frustrating and confusing."

Sarah decided to talk to her doctor about her symptoms. Together, they discussed hormone replacement therapy (HRT) as an option, but Sarah was hesitant due to the potential risks she had heard about. Instead, she focused on making lifestyle changes.

"I started practicing yoga and meditation every morning. It was like a lifeline for me. Slowly, I began to feel more grounded and at peace with the changes happening in my body. I also made sure to eat a balanced diet, cutting out a lot of processed foods, and I started walking every day."

Over time, Sarah's hot flashes became less frequent, and her emotional well-being improved. Today, Sarah feels stronger than ever. "I've learned to embrace this phase of my life. It's not always easy, but I feel more confident and empowered to handle whatever comes my way."

2. Tina's Story: From Sleepless Nights to Restful Sleep

Tina, 48, began experiencing sleep disturbances around the time her periods started becoming irregular. At first, she thought it was just stress from work and personal life. But after several months of restless nights, she realized it might be perimenopause.

"I couldn't sleep for more than two hours at a time," Tina shares. "I'd wake up drenched in sweat, with my heart racing.

I was exhausted during the day and felt like I couldn't function properly."

Tina's doctor suggested she try a few natural remedies before considering medications. "I started taking magnesium before bed, and I made sure to avoid caffeine in the afternoon," Tina explains. "I also started using a cooling pillow and keeping the room temperature lower at night. That made a huge difference."

Within a few weeks, Tina noticed a significant improvement in her sleep. "I'm sleeping much better now, and I feel more energized during the day. I still have occasional nights where I wake up, but it's nothing like before."

Tina's story is a great reminder that small lifestyle adjustments can have a powerful impact on managing symptoms like sleep disturbances. It's not about finding one magic solution; it's about making choices that support your overall health.

3. Maria's Story: Finding Balance in Body and Mind

Maria, 55, had always been active and in good shape. However, as she entered menopause, she noticed a significant change in her body—especially in her weight. "I've always been someone who took care of my body, but during menopause, it felt like no matter how hard I worked out, I couldn't maintain my weight. I was frustrated."

Maria realized that menopause had impacted her metabolism, and she needed to adjust her approach to fitness and nutrition. She worked with a nutritionist who helped her understand how her body's needs had changed.

"I learned to focus on a balanced diet with more whole foods—especially lean proteins and vegetables—and I made sure to stay hydrated. I also shifted my workout routine to focus on strength training and cardio, which helped build muscle and support my metabolism."

Maria's story highlights an important part of menopause: the changes to metabolism and body composition. "It's not about getting back to how I was before; it's about finding what works for my body now."

4. Linda's Story: Strengthening Relationships Through Menopause

Linda, 60, had a very different experience with menopause, one that involved not just physical changes but emotional ones, too. Her partner, Mark, had never fully understood what she was going through, which created tension in their relationship. Linda felt that her moods and symptoms were putting a strain on their marriage.

"I was snapping at him all the time, and I could see how confused and frustrated he was. We were both struggling," Linda recalls.

She decided to have an honest conversation with Mark about menopause and the challenges she was facing. "Once I opened up to him about how I was feeling—about the hot flashes, the mood swings, and the exhaustion—he was incredibly supportive. We even went to a couple of therapy sessions to better understand what we were both going through."

Mark now helps Linda manage her symptoms by being understanding and encouraging her to take breaks when she needs them. "We've found a new rhythm together. It's not perfect, but I feel like we're a team again."

Linda's story is a powerful reminder of the importance of communication and support, both with a partner and with others in your life. Having those tough conversations can strengthen relationships and reduce the emotional burden of menopause.

5. Joan's Story: Empowered by Knowledge and Support

Joan, 50, felt lost when she first started noticing signs of perimenopause. Her periods were irregular, she was constantly fatigued, and her mood felt all over the place. At first, she didn't know where to turn for help.

"I had no idea what was happening to me. I felt so alone," Joan admits. "It wasn't until I reached out to a support group for women going through menopause that things started to change."

In the support group, Joan connected with other women who were going through similar experiences. "I learned so much from the group. Women shared their stories and advice, and I realized I wasn't alone. It made me feel more empowered to take control of my health."

Joan also consulted with her doctor, who recommended a combination of diet changes, exercise, and stress management techniques. "I feel so much better now. I still have some tough days, but I now have the tools and support I need to handle them."

Joan's story is an inspiring example of how connecting with others can make a world of difference. By reaching out for support, Joan was able to find a sense of community and gain the knowledge she needed to navigate menopause with confidence.

Lessons Learned – Wisdom from Women Who've Been There

Menopause is often described as a journey, but what exactly do we learn along the way? As women move through perimenopause, menopause, and postmenopause, they discover things about themselves, their bodies, and their lives that they never expected. In this chapter, we'll reflect on some of the key lessons women have learned during their menopause transitions. These lessons come from women who've faced challenges head-on and have found ways to thrive in spite of them.

This is not just a collection of advice—it's a tapestry of lived experiences, each one a valuable thread of wisdom. The lessons shared here are meant to help guide you as you navigate your own journey with confidence and self-compassion.

1. It's Okay to Ask for Help

The first lesson many women learn during menopause is that they don't have to do it alone. This journey can be full of physical and emotional challenges—hot flashes, fatigue, mood swings, sleep disturbances—and it can feel overwhelming. But one common theme from the stories of women who've successfully navigated menopause is the importance of asking for support.

Clara, 54, shares, "I thought I could handle everything on my own. But when the mood swings got really bad, and I couldn't sleep at night, I realized I needed help. I spoke with my doctor, but I also reached out to my friends and family. It made such a difference."

Clara's experience is a reminder that seeking help isn't a sign of weakness. In fact, it's one of the strongest things you can do. Whether it's talking to your partner, a friend, or a healthcare provider, asking for help can lead to better solutions and a lighter load.

2. Embrace Your New Body, Even with the Changes

As your body goes through menopause, it will change in ways that might feel unexpected. Many women find that they gain weight more easily, their skin feels different, or they experience new aches and pains. It's normal to feel frustrated by these changes, but a key lesson learned by many is to accept and embrace the body you have now, rather than focusing on the one you used to have.

Sue, 58, struggled with weight gain during menopause and says, "I was so hard on myself at first. I wanted to look the same as I did in my 30s. But eventually, I had to accept that my body was changing—and that was okay. I'm still strong and capable, just in a different way."

Sue's story illustrates an important lesson: our bodies are constantly evolving, and menopause is just another phase of that process. The more you can embrace these changes and treat your body with care, the better you'll feel. Focus on strength, vitality, and health, rather than appearance.

3. Prioritize Self-Care—It's Not Selfish, It's Necessary

One of the most important lessons women learn during menopause is the value of self-care. The demands of family, work, and life can often push women to put their own needs last, but menopause is the time to shift that mindset. Taking care of yourself is not selfish—it's essential for your well-being.

Lena, 50, explains, "I always put everyone else first—my kids, my husband, my job. But I started feeling run-down, and it was affecting my health. When I finally made time for myself, even just a few minutes each day, I felt more balanced and happier."

Self-care during menopause can look different for everyone. For some, it might mean taking time for a quiet walk, journaling, or practicing yoga. For others, it could be as simple as getting enough sleep, eating nourishing foods, or saying "no" when needed. The key is recognizing that taking care of your mental, emotional, and physical health is the foundation for navigating this transition with grace.

4. You Don't Have to Choose Between Natural and Medical Treatments

Throughout the menopause journey, women often feel torn between using natural remedies or turning to medical treatments like Hormone Replacement Therapy (HRT). The lesson here is that you don't have to pick one or the other. Many women find that a combination of both works best for them, depending on their symptoms and personal preferences.

Emma, 56, reflects, "At first, I was all about natural remedies. I took herbal supplements and focused on diet changes. But when my hot flashes became unbearable, I decided to try HRT. I was worried about the risks, but my doctor helped me understand the benefits and how to manage it safely. I feel much more balanced now."

Emma's experience shows that menopause care doesn't have to be one-size-fits-all. It's about finding the right approach for you, with guidance from your healthcare provider. And remember, what works for someone else might not work for you—and that's perfectly okay.

5. Understand That Your Mental Health Matters Too

Hormonal changes during menopause can affect more than just your body—they can also impact your mental health. Anxiety, depression, and mood swings are common, but many women are surprised by the emotional rollercoaster they experience.

Rebecca, 57, recalls, "I had no idea how much menopause would affect my emotions. I felt anxious all the time and didn't know why. It wasn't until I talked to my therapist that I understood how the hormonal shifts were affecting me."

Rebecca's story highlights an important lesson: mental health is just as important as physical health during menopause. If you're struggling emotionally, seeking support from a therapist or counselor can be incredibly helpful. Talking to someone who understands the challenges of menopause can make a world of difference.

6. Patience Is Key—This Is a Process, Not a Sprint

One of the hardest lessons for many women is accepting that menopause is not something you can rush through. It's a process that may take several years, and each woman's timeline is different. Being patient with yourself is essential as you move through the different stages of menopause.

Sophia, 60, reflects, "At first, I was so impatient. I wanted to be done with hot flashes, mood swings, and sleepless nights. But I realized that this is just part of the journey. I had to stop rushing through it and learn to embrace the changes as they came."

Sophia's insight speaks to the importance of patience. Menopause isn't something you "get over" quickly, and it's important to give yourself grace throughout the process. Accept that it will take time, and celebrate the small victories along the way.

7. Connect with Other Women

Finally, one of the most powerful lessons women learn is the importance of connection. Menopause can feel isolating, but it doesn't have to be. Finding a community of women who understand what you're going through can provide comfort, camaraderie, and practical advice.

Jennifer, 53, says, "I started attending a menopause support group, and it was a game-changer. Hearing other women's stories made me feel less alone. I realized that what I was going through was normal, and I didn't have to go through it in silence."

Jennifer's experience reinforces the value of support networks. Whether through a formal support group, online forums, or informal conversations with friends, connecting with others who are experiencing similar challenges can offer reassurance and a sense of solidarity.

The menopause journey is unique for each woman, but the lessons learned along the way are universal. Whether it's seeking help when needed, embracing your new body, prioritizing self-care, or learning to be patient, these lessons provide valuable tools to guide you through this phase of life with confidence.

Remember, menopause is not a destination—it's a transition. And with each step, you gain more insight into yourself, your body, and your strength. Trust in your own wisdom, and take this journey one day at a time. You've got this.

Chapter 7
Building a Supportive Community During Menopause

Menopause can often feel like a personal and private journey, but it doesn't have to be one that you face alone. One of the most powerful ways to navigate menopause with strength and confidence is by building a supportive community around you. Sharing your experiences with others who understand can provide comfort, reduce feelings of isolation, and offer practical advice.

In this chapter, we will explore why a supportive community is so important during menopause, and how you can find or build one for yourself. Whether it's through peer support groups, online communities, or local meet-ups, having others to lean on can make all the difference.

Why Building a Supportive Community Matters

During menopause, women can experience a wide range of physical, emotional, and psychological changes. These changes can sometimes feel overwhelming and isolating. It's not uncommon to feel like no one truly understands what you're going through. But here's the good news: **you are not alone.**

Having a community that supports you can help you:

1. **Feel Less Isolated**: Menopause can be a solitary experience if you don't have others to talk to. But

when you connect with other women who are going through similar changes, it creates a sense of shared experience and understanding. You realize that what you're feeling is normal, and it helps you feel less alone in the journey.
2. **Gain Practical Advice**: Peer support groups often provide practical tips for managing symptoms. Whether it's advice on sleep, hot flashes, or emotional changes, other women's insights can be incredibly helpful. You might learn about resources, treatments, or strategies that you haven't considered.
3. **Boost Your Confidence**: When you hear others share their challenges and successes, it reminds you that menopause is a transition that can be handled with grace and resilience. The support of others can help you embrace this phase of life with confidence.
4. **Offer Emotional Support**: Sometimes, just having someone to listen to you is all you need. A supportive community can provide emotional reassurance when you're feeling down, frustrated, or anxious. Knowing that others understand can help you feel validated and heard.

How to Find Support During Menopause

There are several ways you can find a community to support you during menopause. Whether you prefer in-person connections or online groups, there's an option for everyone. Here are some practical suggestions:

1. Peer Support Groups

Peer support groups are one of the most direct ways to connect with others who are experiencing similar menopause challenges. These groups often meet in person, either in your local community or at healthcare centers, libraries, or community centers. They may be organized by a healthcare provider, a nonprofit organization, or even a local wellness center.

Why Peer Support Groups Work:

- **Shared Experience**: Everyone in the group is experiencing similar symptoms, so there's an immediate understanding and empathy.
- **Safe Space**: These groups offer a non-judgmental space where you can talk openly about what you're going through.
- **Accountability**: Many groups offer ongoing support and check-ins, which can keep you on track with managing your health during menopause.

Finding a Group Near You:

- Ask your healthcare provider or local wellness centers if they know of any peer support groups in your area.
- Many nonprofit organizations dedicated to women's health, such as the North American Menopause Society (NAMS), also offer information on local support groups.

2. Online Communities

If you prefer the flexibility of connecting from home, online communities can be a fantastic option. These communities can range from private Facebook groups to forums specifically for women going through menopause. They allow you to share experiences, ask questions, and get advice from women all over the world.

Why Online Communities Work:

- **24/7 Accessibility:** You can connect with others anytime, whether it's during the day or in the middle of the night when insomnia strikes.
- **Diverse Perspectives:** Online groups offer a variety of perspectives and experiences from women of different backgrounds, ages, and locations.
- **Anonymity:** If you're hesitant about talking openly, many online communities offer the option to be anonymous, which can make it easier to share personal experiences.

How to Find Online Communities:

- Search for menopause-related groups on social media platforms like Facebook, Reddit, or Instagram.
- Websites like Menopause Matters or the American Menopause Society also provide online resources and forums for women.
- Consider joining online workshops or webinars that focus on menopause. These events can connect you to others and offer valuable information.

3. Local Meet-Ups

Sometimes, meeting people face-to-face can feel more personal and supportive. Local meet-ups can offer a great way to connect with others in your area who are going through menopause. Websites like Meetup.com can help you find or start a group of women who want to meet up and share their experiences.

Why Meet-Ups Work:

- **In-person Connections:** Being in the same room as others gives you the opportunity to form deeper connections.
- **Social Support:** Beyond just discussing menopause, meet-ups can become social events where you build friendships that extend beyond health discussions.
- **Community Engagement:** These meet-ups help create a sense of community, which can combat feelings of isolation.

How to Get Started:

- Check Meetup.com or similar websites to see if there are existing menopause or women's health groups in your area.
- If you don't find anything, consider starting your own group. You can gather women who are interested in connecting, sharing, and supporting each other.

Benefits of Sharing Your Experience

When you share your story with others, whether in person or online, you give yourself a voice and an opportunity to reflect on your experiences. But it's not just about talking—it's about listening, too. Listening to the experiences of other women can be just as valuable as sharing your own. Here are some of the benefits of sharing your menopause journey:

1. **Relief from Uncertainty:** Talking about your symptoms with others who understand can bring clarity and relief. When you hear that someone else is experiencing the same things, it helps validate your own feelings.
2. **Empowerment:** Knowing that you're part of a larger community of women who are navigating similar challenges can empower you to take control of your health. By sharing information, advice, and support, you help each other build strength and confidence.
3. **Learn New Ideas:** You may discover new ways to manage your symptoms, from diet tips to stress-relief strategies, that you hadn't considered before. Everyone has different tools in their toolbox, and sharing your experiences broadens your options.
4. **Increased Understanding:** Sharing your experiences also helps increase awareness about menopause. It may even help break the stigma surrounding this natural phase of life, making it easier for future generations to embrace menopause with open arms.

How to Create Your Own Support Network

If you're struggling to find a supportive community, don't be afraid to take the initiative. Starting your own support group, either in-person or online, can be a rewarding experience. Here's how to begin:

- **Reach Out:** Start by reaching out to friends, family members, or acquaintances who might be going through menopause or who could offer support. Ask if they'd be interested in joining a group.
- **Set a Goal:** Decide what your group will focus on. It could be general menopause support, or it could

focus on specific areas like sleep, exercise, or nutrition.
- **Keep It Positive:** Make sure your group is a place of positivity, where everyone can share freely without judgment.
- **Stay Consistent:** Consistency is key to building a strong community. Whether you meet monthly or have weekly online discussions, make sure there's regular engagement.

Together, We're Stronger

Building a supportive community during menopause isn't just about feeling heard—it's about thriving together. Whether you find your support group online, at a local meet-up, or by creating your own community, the key is connection. By sharing your experiences and learning from others, you can face menopause with confidence, knowing that you have a network of women who understand and support you.

No one should face menopause alone. Reach out, connect, and build the supportive community that you deserve. Together, we're stronger.

How Family and Friends Can Play a Supportive Role During Menopause

Menopause is a time of great change, both physically and emotionally. While this transition is a deeply personal experience, it's one that can benefit greatly from the support of family and friends. The right kind of support—whether it's listening, understanding, or offering help—can make navigating menopause much easier. In this chapter, we will explore how your loved ones can play a crucial role in this journey and how you can communicate your needs to create a positive, understanding environment.

Why Support from Family and Friends Matters

Menopause can bring about many challenges, such as hot flashes, sleep disturbances, mood swings, and changes in energy levels. These symptoms can sometimes feel overwhelming, especially when you're trying to maintain your regular routine. That's where your family and friends come in. They can provide emotional and practical support that can make the process smoother.

Here's why their support is so important:

- **Emotional Comfort**: Menopause can affect your emotions, causing mood swings, anxiety, or even sadness. Having someone to talk to can help you process these feelings and feel more at ease.
- **Physical Support**: As physical symptoms, like fatigue or joint pain, arise, having family members help with tasks or simply offer encouragement can help ease the load.
- **Increased Understanding**: A supportive environment allows you to feel understood, rather than misunderstood or isolated. It encourages open communication about what you're experiencing, which is essential during this phase of life.

How to Talk to Family and Friends About Menopause

The first step in gaining support from your family and friends is letting them know what you're going through. However, this can sometimes feel challenging, especially if menopause is a topic that hasn't been openly discussed in your circle before. Here are some ways you can initiate conversations and help your loved ones understand:

1. Start the Conversation Early

Don't wait until you're overwhelmed by symptoms to bring up menopause. By starting the conversation early, you set the stage for understanding and support. Explain that menopause is a natural process, not something to be embarrassed about, and that the symptoms can vary from person to person.

Tip: Choose a quiet time when everyone is relaxed and open to discussion. You can begin by sharing a little about what menopause is, what changes you might experience, and how these changes can affect your mood, energy levels, and daily life.

2. Share Your Symptoms and Needs Clearly

Be open about the specific symptoms you are experiencing. This could include hot flashes, sleep problems, fatigue, or mood swings. When you communicate clearly about what you're going through, your loved ones are better equipped to offer the support you need.

For example, you might say, "I've been having hot flashes that make it hard for me to sleep, and I might need some quiet time in the evening to relax." Or, "I've been feeling a little overwhelmed and could use some help with household tasks."

Tip: Use "I" statements to communicate your needs. For example, "I'm feeling tired" or "I need some space to rest." This avoids sounding like you're blaming anyone and makes it easier for your loved ones to understand your needs.

3. Encourage Empathy and Understanding

Encourage your family and friends to educate themselves about menopause. The more they understand, the more empathy and support they will be able to offer. Suggest books, articles, or websites they can explore, or share your own experiences to give them a clearer idea of what you're going through.

Tip: Ask them to listen without offering solutions right away. Sometimes, you just need someone to hear you out and provide emotional validation rather than trying to fix the situation.

Practical Ways Family and Friends Can Offer Support

Now that you've shared your experience, here are some practical ways your loved ones can support you during menopause:

1. Emotional Support

One of the best things family and friends can do is to listen to your feelings and offer emotional support. Whether it's talking through tough moments or offering reassuring words, having someone who listens without judgment can be incredibly comforting.

Tip: Let your loved ones know how they can support you emotionally. For example, you might ask, "When I'm feeling stressed or irritable, can we sit down together and talk about it?" or "It would help if you could just check in with me every now and then to see how I'm feeling."

2. Help with Household Tasks

If you're feeling particularly drained or dealing with physical symptoms like joint pain, household tasks can become overwhelming. Ask for help with chores, cooking, or other responsibilities when you need it.

Tip: If you're not ready to ask for help directly, consider creating a list of tasks that can be shared or rotated. Having a clear plan can reduce stress and make it easier for others to pitch in.

3. Create a Comfortable Environment

Menopause can bring physical discomfort, such as hot flashes or night sweats. Your family can help by making your home environment more comfortable. This might mean adjusting the thermostat, setting up a relaxing space for you to unwind, or making sure there's plenty of water available to stay hydrated.

Tip: Let your family know that small changes, like having a fan nearby or keeping extra blankets for colder nights, can make a big difference in how you feel.

4. Encouragement for Self-Care

Menopause can take a toll on your mental and physical health. Your family can encourage you to take time for self-care, whether it's taking a walk, practicing yoga, reading a book, or simply taking a relaxing bath.

Tip: Ask your family to help remind you to prioritize self-care. For example, you might say, "I've been feeling really stressed lately. Can you encourage me to take a few breaks throughout the day?" or "It would be helpful if you could remind me to get outside for some fresh air."

Setting Boundaries and Managing Expectations

During menopause, it's important to establish boundaries with family and friends. While you want to maintain connections, you also need to prioritize your own health and well-being. This may mean saying no to certain activities or taking more time to rest.

Tip: Don't feel guilty for setting boundaries. Be clear about your limits and communicate them respectfully. For example, "I would love to help out, but I'm feeling really tired right now. Can we plan for another time?"

Creating a Supportive Environment Together

Menopause is a journey, and it's a journey that is made easier with the support of your family and friends. Open communication, empathy, and practical help can make this transition smoother and less stressful. By talking about your needs, sharing your experiences, and encouraging understanding, you can create a positive, supportive environment that helps you embrace this phase of life with confidence.

Remember, you don't have to face menopause alone. With the support of those who care about you, you can navigate these changes with grace, strength, and resilience.

Chapter 8
Creating Your Personal Action Plan for Managing Menopause

Menopause is a unique experience for every woman, and managing its symptoms effectively requires a personalized approach. This chapter will guide you through the process of creating an action plan that combines both natural remedies and medical treatments to suit your individual needs. By following a step-by-step approach, you'll be able to take control of your health and navigate this stage of life with confidence.

Step 1: Understanding Your Symptoms and Needs

Before you can create a personalized action plan, it's important to take a step back and assess what symptoms you are experiencing and how they affect your daily life. Menopause symptoms can vary widely from person to person. Common symptoms include:

- Hot flashes and night sweats
- Sleep disturbances
- Mood swings, anxiety, or irritability
- Fatigue and low energy
- Weight gain or changes in metabolism
- Vaginal dryness or discomfort
- Memory lapses or concentration issues

Action Steps:

1. **Keep a Symptom Journal:** Over the next week or two, track your symptoms. Write down when they occur, their intensity, and how they affect your mood or daily activities. This will help you identify patterns and pinpoint which symptoms are most disruptive to your life.
2. **Assess Your Lifestyle:** Think about how your current lifestyle (diet, exercise, sleep habits) might be affecting your symptoms. Are you getting enough sleep? Are you eating well? Do you exercise regularly? This reflection will help you decide what areas to focus on.

Step 2: Determine Your Treatment Options

Once you've identified your symptoms and lifestyle factors, you can begin to explore your treatment options. There are two main approaches: **natural remedies** and **medical treatments**. It's important to remember that you don't have to choose one over the other; combining both can often be the most effective approach.

Natural Remedies:

These are often the first choice for women seeking a gentler approach to symptom management. Many natural remedies can help relieve symptoms without the use of medications. Some options include:

- **Herbal Remedies:** Some herbs, such as black cohosh, red clover, and sage, have been shown to

help with hot flashes and mood swings. However, it's important to consult with your healthcare provider before trying any herbs to ensure they're safe for you.
- **Dietary Changes:** A balanced diet rich in fruits, vegetables, whole grains, and lean proteins can help manage weight gain, boost energy, and stabilize mood. Foods like soy, flaxseed, and chickpeas may also help balance hormones naturally.
- **Mind-Body Practices:** Yoga, meditation, and deep breathing exercises can help reduce stress and improve mood swings and anxiety. Regular practice can also improve sleep and reduce hot flashes.

Medical Treatments:

If your symptoms are severe or not improving with natural remedies, medical treatments may be necessary. Common medical treatments for menopause symptoms include:

- **Hormone Replacement Therapy (HRT):** HRT is often recommended for women who have severe hot flashes, vaginal dryness, and other significant symptoms. It involves replacing the hormones that are decreasing during menopause.
- **Non-hormonal Medications:** If HRT isn't right for you, there are other options such as antidepressants or medications that help with hot flashes and night sweats.
- **Vaginal Estrogen:** For vaginal dryness and discomfort, a topical form of estrogen can be applied directly to the area to relieve symptoms.

Action Steps:

1. **Discuss Options with Your Healthcare Provider:** It's essential to talk with your doctor or healthcare provider about both natural remedies and medical treatments. They can help you decide what will work best for your symptoms and health history.
2. **Research and Evaluate:** Use reliable sources, such as books, research papers, and trusted websites, to learn more about both natural remedies and medical treatments. Take notes on the pros and cons of each option.

Step 3: Set Realistic Goals and Prioritize Self-Care

Creating a personalized action plan isn't just about choosing treatments—it's also about setting goals and prioritizing self-care. Lifestyle changes can play a significant role in managing menopause symptoms, and self-care practices are essential for your overall well-being.

Action Steps:

1. **Set Symptom Reduction Goals:** Based on your symptom journal, set realistic goals for symptom reduction. For example, if hot flashes are disrupting your sleep, your goal might be to reduce their frequency or intensity over the next three months.
2. **Develop Healthy Habits:**
    - **Exercise:** Incorporating regular physical activity into your routine can improve your energy, reduce hot flashes, and boost your mood. Aim for at least 30 minutes of

- moderate exercise (like walking, swimming, or yoga) 3-5 days a week.
  - **Sleep:** Good sleep hygiene is crucial. Establish a regular sleep schedule, limit caffeine, and create a relaxing bedtime routine to help you sleep better.
  - **Stress Management:** Regular meditation, mindfulness, and relaxation techniques can help manage stress, which can worsen symptoms like hot flashes and anxiety.
3. **Balance Natural and Medical Approaches:** If you're using both natural remedies and medical treatments, make sure you balance them carefully. For example, you might start by trying herbal remedies, and if they're not effective, you can add in medications. Your healthcare provider can help you manage this balance.

Step 4: Review and Adjust Regularly

As menopause is a natural and ongoing process, your needs may change over time. It's important to regularly review your action plan and make adjustments as needed.

Action Steps:

1. **Regular Check-ins:** Every few months, revisit your symptom journal to see how your symptoms are evolving. Are your current remedies working? Are new symptoms emerging? Adjust your plan accordingly.
2. **Evaluate Your Progress:** Consider how well you're managing symptoms like hot flashes, sleep disturbances, and mood swings. Are you achieving

the goals you set? If not, try tweaking your plan. For example, if a dietary change hasn't made a big impact, consider increasing your physical activity or exploring additional medical treatments.
3. **Consult Your Healthcare Provider**: Make regular appointments with your healthcare provider to evaluate your progress and adjust treatments. They can offer support, new options, and expert guidance.

Step 5: Focus on the Bigger Picture

Menopause is not just about managing symptoms—it's also about embracing a new phase of life. Your action plan should include goals that reflect your long-term well-being. This might include focusing on mental health, maintaining a strong social network, and taking time for personal growth.

Action Steps:

1. **Nurture Relationships**: Building a strong support system can help you feel more empowered and understood. Whether it's friends, family, or support groups, staying connected with others is essential.
2. **Prioritize Self-Care**: Continue to make self-care a priority. This can include enjoying hobbies, pursuing new interests, or simply taking time to relax and rejuvenate.
3. **Stay Positive**: Menopause can be challenging, but it's also an opportunity for personal growth and change. With the right plan in place, you can navigate this transition with confidence, embracing the wisdom and strength that comes with this phase of life.

Monitoring the Effectiveness of Treatments and Lifestyle Changes

Making changes to manage menopause can be empowering, but knowing how well these changes are working is just as important. Whether you're trying new treatments, making lifestyle changes, or incorporating natural remedies, tracking your progress is key to understanding what's helping—and what might need adjustment. This chapter will guide you through practical ways to monitor the effectiveness of your treatments and lifestyle changes, helping you make informed decisions and stay encouraged throughout your menopause journey.

Step 1: Keep a Symptom Journal

One of the most helpful ways to track how treatments and lifestyle changes are working is by keeping a symptom journal. This simple tool allows you to note any symptoms you experience, their intensity, and when they occur. By tracking symptoms over time, you can spot patterns and determine which treatments are making a difference.

What to Track:

- **Common Menopause Symptoms:** Hot flashes, night sweats, sleep disturbances, mood changes, anxiety, irritability, fatigue, weight gain, vaginal dryness, and memory lapses.
- **Intensity:** For each symptom, rate its severity on a scale of 1 to 10, with 1 being minimal and 10 being

very intense. This helps you see how your symptoms change over time.
- **Timing:** Record when symptoms occur. Are they worse at certain times of day? Are they connected to specific activities, foods, or stressors?
- **Treatments Used:** Note what remedies or treatments you've tried (e.g., herbal supplements, exercise, HRT, or meditation) and how they make you feel.

Practical Tip:

Try setting aside 5 minutes at the end of each day to fill in your journal. It doesn't need to be complicated—just quick notes on your symptoms and any treatments or lifestyle changes you've implemented that day.

Step 2: Set Realistic Goals

When monitoring progress, it's important to set clear, realistic goals for yourself. These goals will serve as benchmarks, so you know what to expect and can measure how well your treatments and changes are working.

Examples of Goals:

- **Symptom Reduction:** "I want to reduce the frequency of hot flashes from 6 times a day to 2 times a day within the next month."
- **Improved Sleep:** "I want to improve my sleep by falling asleep within 30 minutes and staying asleep for at least 6 hours a night by the end of this month."
- **Stress Management:** "I want to feel calmer and more relaxed after 10 minutes of meditation daily for the next two weeks."

Practical Tip:

Keep your goals simple and attainable. Menopause is a gradual process, and small improvements can be powerful. Aim for progress, not perfection. Review your goals every 2-4 weeks and adjust as needed.

Step 3: Monitor Your Lifestyle Changes

Lifestyle changes such as diet, exercise, and stress management can significantly impact how you feel during menopause. Tracking these changes helps you see what works best for you.

What to Track:

- **Exercise Routine:** Are you exercising regularly? Note the type of exercise (e.g., walking, yoga, strength training) and how often you do it. How does your body feel afterward?
- **Diet:** Keep track of your meals and snacks. Are you eating balanced meals with plenty of fruits, vegetables, whole grains, and lean protein? Are you avoiding foods that trigger symptoms like caffeine, spicy foods, or alcohol?
- **Sleep Patterns:** Record your sleep habits, including the time you go to bed, the time you wake up, and any wakeful periods during the night. Are you feeling more rested or still waking up tired?
- **Stress Levels:** How often are you practicing relaxation techniques like meditation or deep breathing? Do you feel more relaxed or still stressed?

Practical Tip:

Use an app or a simple notebook to track your exercise, meals, sleep, and stress levels. After a week or two, review what's working well and what might need adjustment. If you're feeling more energized or sleeping better, your changes are likely having a positive effect.

Step 4: Evaluate the Effectiveness of Treatments

As you begin to try different treatments, whether they are natural remedies, medical treatments like HRT, or alternative therapies, it's important to assess how well they are working for you. While it's tempting to expect quick fixes, many treatments take time to show results.

What to Evaluate:

- **Symptom Relief:** Are the treatments helping to reduce the frequency or intensity of your symptoms? Track specific improvements, such as fewer hot flashes, better sleep, or less mood instability.
- **Side Effects:** Are you experiencing any new symptoms or side effects from your treatment? For example, HRT can sometimes cause bloating or headaches. Make a note of these so you can discuss them with your healthcare provider.
- **Overall Well-Being:** Do you feel better in general? Are you less fatigued, more positive, or more engaged in your daily life?

Practical Tip:

If you are using a combination of treatments, it may take several weeks to see noticeable changes. Be patient and keep a record of any positive or negative changes you experience. If you don't notice any improvements after a few months, it may be time to reassess your approach.

Step 5: Adjust Your Plan as Needed

Your menopause journey is unique, and as time goes on, your needs may change. It's important to adjust your action plan based on what you're learning from your journal and progress checks. If something isn't working, it might be time to try something else.

How to Adjust:

- **If You're Not Seeing Progress**: If your symptoms aren't improving, it may be time to try a different treatment or make additional lifestyle changes. For example, if you're not seeing improvements with one form of exercise, try a different type, like swimming or Pilates.
- **If Side Effects Appear**: If you experience unwanted side effects from a treatment, talk to your healthcare provider about alternatives or dosage adjustments.
- **If You're Feeling Better**: If you're seeing progress, celebrate it! And, if you're managing symptoms well, your goals might shift. For example, you might decide to focus more on emotional well-being or long-term health.

Practical Tip:

Regularly review your journal and compare it with your goals. If you notice a pattern of progress, it will motivate you to continue with your plan. If things aren't improving, be open to making adjustments.

Step 6: Seek Support and Professional Guidance

As you track your progress, remember that you don't have to do it alone. Talking with a healthcare provider or joining a support group can provide additional insight and guidance. Your doctor can help you evaluate how well your treatment plan is working and offer new options if necessary.

What to Discuss with Your Healthcare Provider:

- **Symptom Changes**: Share your symptom journal with your doctor and discuss whether the treatments you're using are effective.
- **Treatment Adjustments**: Ask your healthcare provider if there are other treatments or combinations that might work better for you.
- **Alternative Therapies**: If you're considering natural remedies, let your doctor know, so they can offer safe and evidence-based suggestions.

Practical Tip:

Consider joining an online or in-person menopause support group. Hearing from others about their experiences and what's worked for them can provide helpful tips and encouragement.

Tracking your progress, evaluating the effectiveness of treatments, and making adjustments are essential parts of managing menopause. By keeping a symptom journal, setting goals, monitoring lifestyle changes, and adjusting your plan as needed, you can stay on top of your health and make the most of your menopause journey. Remember, it's okay to seek professional guidance and support from others. You're not alone in this, and with the right tools and mindset, you can thrive through this transition.

Chapter 9
Embracing the Changes of Menopause

As we reach the end of this guide, it's important to remember one key thing: menopause is not something to fear or endure—it is a natural and powerful part of every woman's life. While the changes that come with perimenopause, menopause, and postmenopause can feel overwhelming at times, they are also an opportunity for growth, renewal, and self-discovery. This chapter will summarize key insights from this book and encourage you to embrace the changes brought by menopause with confidence, self-care, and empowerment.

Understanding the Changes

Throughout this guide, we've explored the physical, emotional, and mental changes that occur during menopause. From hormonal fluctuations to sleep disturbances, hot flashes, and mood changes, these are all part of the journey. You've learned how menopause affects your body and mind, but also how you can manage and even thrive through these changes.

Menopause doesn't mean the end of vitality or joy. In fact, it can mark the beginning of a new chapter in life. This is the time to embrace who you are, take care of your health, and prioritize your well-being.

Empowerment Through Knowledge

One of the most empowering things you can do during menopause is to educate yourself. By understanding what's happening to your body and mind, you can make informed decisions about your health. You've learned about natural remedies, medical treatments, lifestyle changes, and mind-body practices that can help ease your symptoms and improve your quality of life.

Remember, no two experiences of menopause are the same. What works for one woman may not work for another. This is why it's important to listen to your body, track your symptoms, and adjust your approach as needed. Take charge of your health and feel confident in the choices you make.

Self-Care is Key

Self-care is an essential part of navigating menopause. As your body undergoes changes, it's crucial to be kind to yourself. This means making time for relaxation, eating nourishing foods, exercising regularly, and finding joy in the small moments. It also means seeking support from others when you need it—whether through family, friends, support groups, or healthcare providers.

By making self-care a priority, you not only improve your health but also your emotional well-being. Menopause is a time of transformation, and you have the power to shape this experience in a way that works best for you.

Building a Support System

You don't have to go through menopause alone. One of the most powerful ways to thrive during this transition is by building a supportive community. Surround yourself with people who understand and uplift you. Whether it's friends, family, or online groups, connecting with others who are going through the same experience can be incredibly comforting and empowering.

Talking openly about menopause, sharing your challenges, and celebrating your successes with others helps normalize the experience and reduces feelings of isolation. Remember, you're not alone in this journey, and reaching out for support is a sign of strength, not weakness.

Taking Action and Staying Positive

As you move forward, take action to manage your symptoms and embrace your new phase of life. Set realistic goals, track your progress, and adjust your plan when needed. Use the tools and strategies you've learned in this book to feel more confident, healthier, and more in control.

Stay positive, too. Menopause is not the end of your story—it's a new beginning. It's a chance to focus on yourself, your health, and your happiness. With the right mindset, you can not only navigate menopause but also come out of it stronger and more empowered than ever.

Celebrating the Journey

Finally, take a moment to celebrate the incredible journey you've been on. Menopause is a transition, but it's also an opportunity to reflect on everything you've learned and everything you've become. You've made it this far, and you have the tools, knowledge, and strength to continue forward with confidence.

The changes you're going through are a natural part of life, and by embracing them with self-care, support, and empowerment, you can make this phase of life one of your most fulfilling yet.

You Are Strong, You Are Capable, and You Are Not Alone

As you continue your menopause journey, remember that you are strong, capable, and deserving of all the support and care you need. Embrace the changes that come, and let this new chapter be one of growth, joy, and vitality. You've got this, and we are all in this together.

Looking Forward: Embracing the Future with Optimism

As you reach the end of this book, I want to leave you with one powerful thought: **this is just the beginning of a new chapter in your life.** Menopause is a transition, not an end. It's a time to embrace your personal growth, take care of your body and mind, and focus on what truly brings you joy and fulfillment.

Throughout this book, we've explored the changes you might experience during perimenopause, menopause, and postmenopause. We've also discussed strategies to manage those changes—whether through natural remedies, medical treatments, lifestyle adjustments, or emotional support. All of these tools are now part of your toolbox, ready to help you navigate this phase with confidence.

You Are in Control

One of the most empowering things you can take away from this book is the knowledge that you are in control of your own journey. The advice shared here is just that—advice. It's up to you to decide what works best for your body, your health, and your life. You don't have to follow a one-size-fits-all approach. By listening to your body, adjusting your plans when needed, and making informed choices, you are in the driver's seat.

Remember, every woman's menopause experience is unique. What works for one may not work for another. But with the tools, strategies, and knowledge you now have, you can confidently create a plan that works for you. You are the expert in your own life.

New Beginnings, Not an End

Many women feel uncertain or even apprehensive about menopause because it's often framed as the "end of youth" or the "end of vitality." But in reality, it's a new beginning—a time for renewal, personal growth, and rediscovery. Your life doesn't stop here; it evolves. You may find that this new chapter gives you the chance to focus on things that truly matter to you—whether that's taking up new hobbies, strengthening relationships, focusing on your health, or simply enjoying more time for yourself.

Menopause can also bring newfound wisdom, confidence, and a deeper connection to your own body. You may discover that the changes you experience allow you to be more mindful, more in tune with your needs, and more empowered to make decisions that support your well-being.

Optimism for the Future

As you move forward, think of menopause as an opportunity to take charge of your health and happiness. There is so much to look forward to! With the knowledge and strategies from this book, you're not only equipped to handle menopausal symptoms, but you're also positioned to embrace the future with optimism.

You have the power to create a vibrant, fulfilling life at any stage. Your journey doesn't end here—it's just a new chapter filled with possibility. With the support of your family, friends, and the community around you, you can face this time with hope, confidence, and a sense of adventure.

A Future Full of Possibilities

While menopause may come with some challenges, it also brings the opportunity for growth, strength, and new beginnings. There are so many possibilities ahead. Whether it's focusing on your health, exploring new passions, or simply enjoying the freedom that comes with this stage of life, your future is bright.

So, take a deep breath, hold your head high, and step into the next phase of your life with optimism. The strategies you've learned in this book will guide you, but your strength and determination will carry you forward.

You've Got This

In closing, I want you to remember this: You've got this. You are more capable than you realize, and you are not alone on this journey. With the right tools, a positive mindset, and the support of those around you, you can Redefining Midlife and beyond.

Here's to embracing the changes, celebrating the future, and living the best version of yourself. The next chapter of your life holds endless opportunities—so let's step into it with confidence, optimism, and a full heart. The best is yet to come.

Made in the USA
Monee, IL
30 May 2025